The Stress Cure

A Simple 7-Step Plan to

Balance Mood,

Improve Memory,

and Restore Energy

The
Stress
Cure

Vern S. Cherewatenko, M.D.,
and Paul Perry

HarperResource
An Imprint of HarperCollins*Publishers*

HarperCollins books may be purchased for educational, business, or sales promotional use. For information please write: Special Markets Department, HarperCollins Publishers Inc., 10 East 53rd Street, New York, NY 10022.

FIRST EDITION

Printed on acid-free paper

Designed by Ellen Cipriano

Library of Congress Cataloging-in-Publication Data

Cherewatenko, Vern S.
    The stress cure : a simple 7-step plan to balance mood, improve memory, and restore energy / Vern S. Cherewatenko and Paul Perry.
        p. cm.
    Includes bibliographical references and index.
    ISBN 0-06-019825-7
        1. Stress management for women.   2. Medicine, Popular.   3. Stress (Physiology)   4. Stress (Psychology)   I. Perry, Paul, 1950–   II. Title.
    RA778.C423 2003
    155.9'042'082—dc21

                                                        2003047874

03 04 05 06 07 WB/RRD 10 9 8 7 6 5 4 3 2 1

To my patients who entrusted me with their most intimate feelings and emotions—and to those who are still suffering in silence.

Contents

Acknowledgments

It is a difficult task to thank all of the people who were an inspiration in writing *The Stress Cure*. Some gifted pioneers cannot go unmentioned. A debt of gratitude is owed to Hans Selye, M.D., the father of stress research, whose life focus evolved around explaining the physiological symphony that occurs in each of us as we navigate the stress of life; and to Claude Bernard and Walter B. Cannon, the grandfathers of stress research, who dedicated their lives to understanding the wonderment of our internal physiology as it responds to the environment we live in. Appreciation is given to the countless clinicians and researchers who have expanded on these early pioneers and have published scientific articles and medical texts so that more of us can understand the complexities associated with stress, illness, and disease.

The rapid expansion of the field of functional medicine has been a beacon of light in the increasingly frustrating sea of traditional medicine. The warrior of this discipline, Jeffrey Bland, Ph.D., has spent over 25 years educating physicians like myself about the field of orthomolecular medicine. Linus Pauling, Ph.D., Roger Williams, Ph.D., and Abram Hofer, M.D., Ph.D., are credited with giving birth to the fields of molecular medicine, biochemical individuality, and biomolecular psychiatry respectively. The essence of their teachings set the stage for the basis of the phrase "Biology drives behavior." The current and future integration of clinical nutrition, dietary considerations, lifestyle, and environmental management will become the new standard of care for mainstream medicine.

Several individuals and corporations have played an essential part in aiding patients and their health care providers with education, diagnostic, and therapeutic resources. These individuals are international teaching icons and their respective companies provide outstanding educational opportunities for both patients and clinicians. Many thanks to the following individuals for their contributions, dedication, and expertise to the field: Jeffrey Bland, Ph.D., Dan Lukaczer, N.D., Robert Rakowski, D.C., and the staff of the Institute for Functional Medicine; Jeffrey Zavik and Kauley Jones of Immuno Laboratories; The Katke Family of Metagenics, Incorporated; Stephen Merritt and Brad Rachman, D.C., of Great Smokies Diagnostic Laboratories; Bill Downs of InterHealth Nutriceuticals; Christian Renna, D.O., of LifeSpan Medicine; Steve Kaye, M.D., of Lifeline Balance Centers; Kevin Connolly, Ph.D., of River Valley Psychological Associates; Riley Livingston of BioGenesis; Gary Bassett, N.D., Ph.D., of Direct Laboratory Services; Physiologics; Douglas Laboratories; Hernan Acevado, Ph.D., Aldar Bourinbayar, Ph.D.; Soheyla Mousavi, Ph.D.; David MacDonald, D.O.; James Braly, M.D.; Howard Lyman; Mike Gardiner; Jonathan Wright, M.D.; Joseph Pizzorno, N.D.; Michael Murray, N.D.

Before a book is published a multitude of tasks must be completed. From the initial concept through the point of sale, those behind the scenes were instrumental in getting this book into its final shape. I am indebted to Paul Perry for his patience and unique literary expertise and to Mel Morse, M.D., for introducing me to Paul and for opening the door to Harper-Collins. Thanks to Diane Reverand, who believed in the concept and gave it birth, and to Toni Sciarra, our editor at HarperCollins who nurtured the book through to completion. Thanks to Nancy Intrator for her expertise with multiple revisions and her patience with my over-busy schedule. And lastly, to our agent, Nat Sobel, for promoting our work and monitoring its progress.

My staff must be thanked for their outstanding ability to withstand and support the many tasks I juggle as a busy clinician on a daily basis. They have been steadfast at my side to provide the assistance I need in treating patients and dealing with the never-ending needs and fallout from the various projects I am involved with. Abby de La Cruz, my medical assistant and patient care coordinator, and Maryzen Caoagdan, my administrative assistant, deserve medals of honor for their persistent efforts. Special thanks to Lori Swanz for her dedication and devotion to helping patients learn that there is usually a modifiable biological explanation for the uncomfortable behaviors and emotions that they experience on a daily basis. In addition to managing my two corporations, being a nutritional role model, and protecting me from myself, Lori has been vital in helping me teach thousands of people in a variety of formats about stress and DHEA. Thanks to my best buddy, Donald Whittaker, who has listened to my dreams and ideas, for making me and this world a better place, and to James Coffin, who, through his creative artistry, has taught me the virtues of living in the here and now. Last, my sincere appreciation to my family—Jeanine, Rachel, Kelsey, and Megan—who I have caused more stress than they deserve. It is no small challenge to have a physician as a husband and father. Thank you for your patience and understanding over the years—I love you all.

Before You Begin This Book

Complete freedom from stress is death.
HANS SELYE, M.D., PH.D.

This is a book about renewal of body and spirit. It is written for women. This is not because you are the only gender to encounter stress. But in addition to dealing with the everyday demands related to your job, partner, husband, children, finances, environment, and other challenges—not to mention your concerns about the future—there are other factors that make your lives more stressful than those of men.

The primary cause of stress is biological. The way you treat yourself and others is often linked strongly to your levels of various hormones. Hormones are chemical messengers that make you behave and feel certain ways. Ever changing, your hormones play an enormous role in controlling your emotions and almost everything else in your body, from cell growth and sexual development to energy levels, from your response to illness to your interactions with others.

When you were just entering womanhood, you may have felt sexy and powerful. You had more energy and a greater sense of humor. You enjoyed life and looked forward to each new day. Those feelings were due, in large part, to the high levels and the correct balance of hormones circulating throughout your body. But as you have lived, aged, become overwhelmed by stress, or all of the above, the hormones that made you feel energetic, sexy, and in love with life have begun to lose their power.

Regaining that power is what The Stress Cure is all about.

Is This You?

I'll give you an example of the effects of stress and the dramatic potential of The Stress Cure with a patient I will call Rebecca. Your situation may not match hers exactly, but her story will give you an idea of the magnitude of change possible.

Rebecca came to my office complaining of memory loss, periods of confusion, headaches, depression, and general irritability. "I don't know what's wrong," said the 47-year-old. "I just feel like I'm ready to bite someone's head off most of the time. I don't feel like the person I once was. It's as if I'm becoming someone else, and I don't like that person. What is happening to me?" She looked at me, bewildered. "I just don't understand *why* I feel this way."

These are common complaints I hear every day from women I see in my practice who are in need of The Stress Cure. The majority of women experience similar symptoms. They may also be experiencing muscle aches, stomach pain, diarrhea, fatigue, memory loss, confusion, anxiety, difficulty in concentrating, or weight gain. They sense that a larger problem is causing their distinct symptoms, but they don't know what it is. Rebecca was no different.

"Maybe my thyroid isn't working," she suggested. "I've asked other doctors about my thyroid. They test me and tell me everything looks fine, and then they send me on my way."

I asked her to tell me if she frequently felt overwhelmed. Immediately her upper chest and neck began to flush with redness. "Yes, I do," she said, nervously clasping her hands.

"Do you feel as if you have much more to do than you are capable of doing?" I asked.

"Yes, all the time," she said. "Sometimes I feel like I'm losing control of everything."

"What is your energy level? Do you find yourself fatigued a lot?"

"I'm tired all the time. Even when I get a full night's sleep, I feel exhausted."

"Have you felt a decrease in your sex drive?"

"What sex drive?" she replied, sounding as though she was trying to hold back tears. "I don't even know what that is anymore."

"Would it help you to know that you're not alone?" I asked. "This is a problem that affects many women."

Rebecca started to sob. I handed her a tissue and we sat in silence for several seconds.

"I'm sorry," she said. "I don't know what came over me. I'm usually not like this."

"You have nothing to apologize for, Rebecca," I said. "But it seems clear that we're dealing with something a little bigger than just a headache."

"Wow!" she said, exhaling deeply. "I didn't know I had so much bottled up inside."

After Rebecca regained her composure, I explained that her headaches were most likely a direct result of a decreased ability to cope with the daily barrage of stressful events in her life.

"I can help you understand what is going on in your body and in your life to trigger these feelings," I told Rebecca. "There is a biological reason you're feeling this way. I'll help you understand the biochemical imbalance that is occurring inside you. Then we can work together to correct it. I will help you get back to feeling like your old self again."

Just as I explained to Rebecca the series of events that occur in the body when a person is confronted repeatedly with excess stress, so this book will describe those same associations to you in some detail. Chief among the issues—and one that was key in Rebecca's case and in the cases of many women I treat—is this: A primary factor in the physical response to stress is the body's *excess* levels of the hormone cortisol and resulting *low* level of the hormone DHEA (dehydroepiandrosterone), which I call "the hormone of coping."

When under stress, the body releases cortisol, which puts all body systems on high alert to confront the crisis. Too much cortisol can be harmful to the body. Normally, DHEA balances the potentially damaging effects of cortisol. But when the body is under stress, the production of DHEA is suppressed and cortisol levels rise, unchecked. That is why supplemental DHEA, taken in appropriate doses, is the cornerstone of The Stress Cure. You will learn much more about this hormone and its complex interaction with your other hormones in later chapters.

The Magic of DHEA

The most important thing we needed to do for Rebecca was perform blood and saliva tests to determine whether insufficient DHEA was really causing her symptoms. A woman of Rebecca's age should have a DHEA level of 550 ng/dl (nanograms per deciliter of blood). As I suspected, the laboratory reports confirmed that Rebecca's levels of DHEA were nearly zero. Low DHEA is often accompanied by low levels of the hormones estrogen, progesterone, and testosterone. Since they, too, are important to emotional balance, I checked Rebecca's levels of those hormones. They were similarly low.

I prescribed 25 milligrams (mg) of DHEA per day for Rebecca, and I asked her to come see me again in three weeks. At her follow-up visit the change was astounding. The stress was gone from her face, and she was actually smiling as we talked about the last few weeks. "Within three days of taking the DHEA I felt everything inside of me lift," she said. "It was like I had come back from the edge. I feel more in control."

Rebecca went on to tell me that little things didn't bother her anymore. As an example, she described an incident with her young daughter, who had knocked over a glass of juice at the dinner table a week earlier. "That same thing happened a few weeks before I started taking DHEA, and I went ballistic," she said. "This time I asked her to be more careful and helped her clean up the mess. I am completely different." Rebecca was amazed at the change, and so was her husband.

Other things in her life had changed, too. Her headaches had disappeared, as had her frequent fatigue. She reported better concentration, lower levels of anxiety, and no more periods of confusion or memory loss. And she was losing weight for the first time in years.

"It's a strange way to put it, but I feel human again," she said. "There were so many demands on me that I had been feeling like a robot. Now there are still demands, but I'm coping with them differently. I am even enjoying my husband again—if you know what I mean."

I had my lab assistant draw blood again and found that Rebecca's DHEA level was a healthier 120ng/dl. Her estrogen, progesterone, and testosterone levels all had improved as well. She felt the best she had felt in years; she only wished she had learned about DHEA years before.

Going for Total Victory

I could have declared victory at that point and sent Rebecca home. The DHEA had made her feel 80% normal in just a short period of time. But I was still interested in that other 20%.

Even though Rebecca felt better when taking the DHEA, her life was still very demanding. She worked 40 hours a week and commuted an additional 10 hours. Rebecca also cooked, cleaned, washed clothes, helped her children with homework, listened to her husband's complaints about work, paid the household bills, and hoped nothing else would come up to occupy what little extra time she had to herself—"extra time" that usually never occurred.

The Disease of Stressful Living

If she continued to try to deal with so many stressors in her life, Rebecca would backslide. In essence, stress would continue to destroy the positive benefits of DHEA.

"We have to work on other aspects of your life," I told her. "To just take it this far would be to treat the symptoms, but not the disease, of stressful living."

"Where do I start?" she asked.

Together we drew up a partial checklist of stressors in her life:

- In the morning, getting the children up, fed, and dressed; reviewing homework, making lunches, and getting them out the door to go to school on time.
- Getting ready for work and leaving enough time for before-work errands.
- Listening to her boss complain about his life.
- Doing multiple tasks at her job, along with additional tasks assigned to her because she is so "efficient."
- Running errands after work, including buying food for dinner.
- Trying to prepare a nutritious, appealing dinner after a hard day's work.
- Listening to her family complain about dinner.

- Listening to her husband complain about his job and his own stress.
- Cleaning the house, dusting, washing, vacuuming, and restocking the pantry.
- Feeling overwhelmed by sensations of negativity, loneliness, inadequacy, and aging.
- Experiencing physical pains in joints and other areas.
- Feeling mentally and physically tired but not having time for a rest.
- Having aging parents and dealing with sibling stresses surrounding their care.
- Having uncomfortable levels of debt, with no perceived solution other than to work even harder.
- Most important: Having no one listen when she needs emotional support.

"Although DHEA supplementation can help you better cope with these problems, it won't get rid of them," I explained. "As we live life, our body is processing information at lightning speed. When events occur that seem to leave us with less control, our bodies go on guard. It is this sense of being out of control that depletes our energies and contributes to stress. If you learn to identify and classify your stressors, you can begin to take control of them. You will begin to protect and restore your hormone balance, ultimately leading to a healthy mind, body, and spirit."

Regaining Control

Once Rebecca's ability to cope had been boosted by DHEA therapy and her other related hormones were on the rise, she was ready for the behavioral part of the program. The focus of this part of The Stress Cure is to regain a greater level of control over one's life.

"Nutritional supplements, stress management, working on your relationships, exercise, proper nutrition, and getting the proper sleep are all important elements of The Stress Cure," I told Rebecca. "Doing these things won't give you total control over your life, but they will improve your ability to handle life's curveballs."

The "Big Picture" in Medicine

Many patients like Rebecca have lost hope that they will ever feel better because of the inability of traditional medical practitioners to treat the whole patient rather than address individual symptoms. Typically, physicians tend to prescribe a separate medication for each complaint: an anti-inflammatory medication for arthritis, an antidepressant for "the blues," and so on. Fortunately, many of my colleagues are beginning to realize that there is a better way to practice medicine. Doctors like myself, who practice functional medicine, are looking for the bigger picture when it comes to our patients' health. Rather than trying to match a disease process with the latest designer prescription medication, we look at each of our patients as a whole person made up of interconnected organs and body systems that function together. Numerous individual symptoms can often be traced to a single systemic problem that is affecting multiple areas of the body simultaneously.

My Mission

I have introduced hundreds of women to The Stress Cure and helped them balance their lives and manage their stress by influencing both *internal* stressors caused by imbalances in their stress hormones and *external* stressors caused by demanding jobs, husbands, children, and—perhaps most damaging—self-imposed expectations.

Before beginning The Stress Cure, these women felt angry, overwhelmed, defeated, depressed, rejected, overworked, numb, lost, unhappy, unfulfilled, hostile, frustrated, and trapped. Within days of starting The Stress Cure, they felt as though a mysterious veil of gloom had been lifted. "It was like the world had color again," said one patient.

Road Map to Stress Reduction

This book is going to tell you exactly how you, too, can use The Stress Cure to regain control over the sources of stress in your own life.

Since you cannot work on reducing stress unless you understand what causes it, Part I of *The Stress Cure* will tell you all you need to know about stress. Chapter 1 describes the various symptoms and manifestations of stress and stress-related illnesses. You may even recognize yourself in some of the case studies. Chapter 2 explains how biology drives behavior. In it I will explain the medical aspects of stress, discuss the roles of DHEA, cortisol, and other stress-related hormones, and describe some clinical studies on the relationship between stress and various diseases. Chapter 3 presents information on various internal and external stressors that add pressure to our lives.

By the time you get to chapter 4 you'll have a solid grounding in the causes and manifestations of stress. Then it will be time for you to find a pencil and do some soul-searching. Chapter 4 contains The Stress Cure Inventory, a self-assessment to help you evaluate your own level of stress. Please don't let this questionnaire add to your anxiety. The results are for your own private use, and they are meant to help you get the most out of The Stress Cure.

Part II presents The Stress Cure: Seven Steps to De-STRESS

Step 1: **D**ehydroepiandrosterone (DHEA)

For most women, the first step to The Stress Cure is to restore their DHEA levels to normal. This is accomplished through supplements. Appropriate levels of DHEA help your body withstand and respond appropriately to stress.

Step 2: **S**upplemental Nutrition

Stress robs your body of many of its other vital nutrients, in addition to DHEA. Replenishing lost vitamins, minerals, and electrolytes is another important key to overcoming stress. In this chapter you will discover how to replenish these nutrients through the use of supplements.

Step 3: **T**aming the Tiger

Time spent in meditation, yoga, reading, and even taking warm baths can help reduce the stress in your life. Whichever method you choose for "mindful living," this book offers advice on how to do it effectively.

Step 4: **R**ekindling Relationships

Troubled relationships are among the greatest contributors to stress. The Stress Cure will show you some new approaches to regaining the closeness that may be missing in the relationships that are most important to you.

Step 5: Effective Exercising

Exercise is good for our hearts, lungs, muscles, brains, and just about every aspect of our health. It makes sense that exercise should also help our bodies cope with stress. In The Stress Cure we focus on exercising in such a way as to increase energy and mental focus.

Step 6: Sensible Eating

Stress drives many women to the refrigerator. In this book we will focus on dietary and behavioral methods of keeping your emotions from ruling your palate.

Step 7: Sound Sleep

Sleep makes it possible for the body to replenish its resources. Proper sleep habits and a good quality of sleep can help balance the hormones that keep us emotionally stable. This book will offer guidance on how to make sure you get the sleep you need and deserve.

Asking for Help

Often the most difficult hurdle for a patient is admitting that she is over-stressed and needs help. Most of the women who come to my office do not realize that stress is at the root of their problems. They simply do not recognize the relationship between stress and their particular physical complaints.

You have taken the first step in asking for help by opening this book. If you follow the road map, read through the background information, fill out the self-assessment questionnaire, and follow the seven steps to De-STRESS, you will be well on your way to better health and a more fulfilling lifestyle.

What Happened to Rebecca?

Rebecca went from being literally consumed by the demands and stresses of her daily life to being in control of them. How did that happen? Like so many of my other patients, by using the program set forth in this book, Rebecca was able to tackle her stress first on a biochemical level, and then on the physical and psychological levels. The Stress Cure put her back in control of her thoughts, feelings, and actions.

Patients like Rebecca and others you will meet in this book have proven that the chronic condition of stress can be cured. All it takes is the courage to change. It is my profound hope that each and every one of you has the courage to follow my road map to make your way toward greater health, happiness, and control over your lives.

PART I

All about Stress

CHAPTER ONE

"Broken in Pieces All Over"

There are many definitions for stress and for *female* stress. I prefer to keep mine rather simple. I diagnose female stress syndrome when a woman experiences persistent and recurrent feelings of sadness, being overwhelmed, physical exhaustion, emotional and mental exhaustion, extreme anxiety or tension, anger or rage, irritability, or a general feeling of being out of control. It is literally like running out of gas, but in this case the "gas" is the fuel to cope, or the energy women need to deal with life's ever-increasing responsibilities.

Women all over the world suffer more stress in their lives than men. This does not mean that men do not experience stress; nor does it mean that men will not learn from this book. In fact, just the opposite is true.

Faced with levels of stress not previously encountered for such extended periods of time, women are suffering in silence, trying to keep up with the increased demands placed on them. This is especially true of full-time mothers with children under the age of 13. But a study conducted by Roper Starch Worldwide, which covered the United States, Britain, Germany, France, Russia, Hungary, South Africa, Brazil, Argentina, China, India, Indonesia, and the Philippines showed that life is tougher on women across the board:

- More white-collar women feel "superstressed" than their male counterparts.
- More single women feel intense daily stress than single men.

- Divorced or separated women feel far more stress than divorced or separated men.
- Widowed women feel more stressed than widowed men by a margin of almost two to one.

The Picture of Stress

I am always intrigued and moved by the images women use to describe their plight. The following are direct quotes from my patients. They are typical of what my staff and I hear nearly every day. Each of these women is suffering from female stress syndrome, and most of them don't even know it. You can almost feel the passion and desperation in their statements.

- "It feels as though something inside of me is ready to explode."
- "I have almost no power over what I do or say. I feel completely out of control."
- "I find myself lashing out at things, people, and situations that I shouldn't even be upset about."
- "I have waves of fear and panic that don't make sense."
- "I feel like Humpty Dumpty. It is as though I have fallen off a wall and I am broken in pieces all over."
- "I am angry for no reason at all."
- "I feel overwhelmed by everything."
- "I am numb. It is as if I have no good feelings anymore."
- "I feel completely overworked all the time."
- "I can't wake up. I just feel tired constantly."
- "I am short-tempered with everyone in the family—especially my husband—even though he hasn't done anything wrong. I have a great husband and great kids. Sometimes I don't know why they even put up with me."
- "I feel trapped by responsibility."
- "My life has become an emotional roller coaster."
- "I feel taken for granted, and it makes me feel hopeless."
- "I feel alone . . . lost . . . unhappy . . . unfulfilled . . . frustrated."
- "It seems like I yell at my kids all the time. I have no patience."
- "I feel tremendously guilty."
- "I just want to go away."

- "It seems as though no one understands me."
- "No one listens to me."
- "I am not myself—it's as if I'm possessed."
- "I ache all over . . . my body, my mind, my heart."
- "I am always so down in the dumps."
- "I feel as if my life has been taken away. . . . I keep trying to get it back, but I can't seem to feel happy like I used to be."
- "I don't care about sex anymore."

Stress-Related Complaints

When women come to see me, they do not always realize that their problems have stress-based causes. In fact, many are surprised when I mention that stress could be the reason they are experiencing the problems they are having. Many almost reflexively deny that they're under great stress. Keri, a 40-year-old mother of two, insisted that she wasn't under much stress. Then she proceeded to tell me that two years earlier she had had a serious automobile accident. Thankfully, everyone in the car survived. Keri also had experienced the deaths of a colleague and several distant family members within the previous month. For three months she had been averaging only about three hours of interrupted sleep each night. She and her husband were arguing frequently. But she still insisted she was under no stress! Instead, Keri came in complaining of severe headaches that were increasing in intensity. She was fatigued nearly all the time, and her sex drive was nonexistent. Her back, neck, and shoulders were painful to the touch, and she felt as if her upper back was in constant spasm. She tried all of the treatments that her several doctors had prescribed, yet none had made any significant improvement in her health. She felt as if she was losing ground and wanted to find out what was really wrong with her.

Warning Signs

Here are some red-flag complaints, or secondary symptoms, that cause me to suspect that a patient may be suffering from female stress.

Fatigue	Muscle aches
Headaches, migraines	Abnormal throat sensations
Weight gain or loss	Sweating abnormalities

PMS	Heat and/or cold intolerance
Irritability	Low self-esteem
Fluid retention	Light-headedness
Anxiety, panic attacks	Easy bruising
Chest pain, quickened heart rate	Acid indigestion, stomach pains
Hair loss	Flushing
Depression	Cold or blue hands or feet
Decreased memory, confusion	Poor coordination
Decreased sex drive	Hypoglycemia
Unhealthy nails	Abnormal swallowing
Low motivation	Excessively tired after eating
Irritable bowel syndrome	Dry eyes and blurred vision
Insomnia	Hives
Arthritis and joint aches	Itchiness
Decreased concentration	Infertility

Portraits of Stress from My Own Files

Jenny came into my office with a bright smile on her face that belied her complaint. "Doctor," she said in the examining room, "I think I am going crazy."

"You don't look like you are," I said, pulling out a note pad. I wrote down what she said and also how she looked. She was dressed in a business suit and high heels. She was not overweight, but I could tell by the way her clothing fit that she had recently gained a few pounds. I also noted that her smile was beginning to wilt as she talked about herself.

"For a long time I was okay if I stayed really busy," she said. "Lately I feel like I'm not okay at all."

She was an office manager at a large law firm and had recently "gone into a tailspin" when pressure was put on her to find some new secretaries.

"I have become irritable, short-tempered, and intolerant," she said. "I have even tried to convince myself that I have earned the right to be short-tempered with people, but the fact is that I have no control over it."

Lately she had begun to feel very disorganized and forgetful. She thought this might be because she wasn't sleeping well, and she blamed not sleeping well on having stopped exercising. "I am just too tired to exercise," she said. "How's that for a vicious cycle?"

Home used to be a haven for Jenny. "Now everything looks unfinished to me," she said. "The house always seems a mess, even when it's not."

Jenny's irritation with everything had begun to bother her husband. "He seems to be avoiding me these days," she said.

When Jenny logically examined her life, she could find nothing wrong. Still, nothing felt quite right. "It just feels like things are getting worse when they aren't," she said. "Every day gets tougher. I feel guilty, and I don't know why. I feel out of control for no reason. My life seems to be centered around fear, even though I have nothing to be afraid of."

And that, said Jenny, was why she felt like she was going crazy.

Taming of the Shrew

When I first met Mary she was quite agitated. She cut to the chase as soon as I asked her what was wrong.

"I have turned into a shrew," she said. "I don't know what happened. Life has always been stressful. My husband and I both make good money, but we have two children, and we do wonder where it goes every month. It has been a challenge to get by, but it has also been fun. In the last year, though, life has stopped being fun. Instead, it has turned into hell."

"Did anything in particular happen?" I asked.

"No. That's the funny thing," she said. "All of a sudden I can't get anything done. I am exhausted all the time. I usually sleep only about four or five hours a night."

Mary started feeling "like a different person" about six months before coming to see me. At first there were subtle changes, like not sleeping enough and feeling constantly tired. Then she began snapping at her coworkers. She became short with them when they asked what was wrong.

"I have no control over my emotions," she said, a common refrain among women with female stress syndrome. "I have been frustrating everyone around me, and I am ashamed and embarrassed, which makes it even harder for me to cope with all this. Still, it seems there's nothing I can do about it."

"I hear people say that a lot," I said.

"Do you hear them say that they are losing their memory?" Mary asked. "Since this started, my memory has gotten worse and worse. I am beginning to wonder if I am developing Alzheimer's."

"That's highly unlikely," I assured her.

Oh, Susannah!

When Susannah walked into my office, she was thin and pale, with dark circles under her eyes. She had made an appointment to see me because she had been having digestive problems. She told me she always felt as though she had an upset stomach, and it seemed as though there was a lump in her throat. The mere act of eating exhausted her.

"Just thinking about having to prepare a meal tires me out," Susannah said. "I used to love to cook. Now I seem to be all thumbs in the kitchen. I drop things. I can't measure the ingredients. I make mistakes. I get so angry at myself when things don't turn out right. I can't even scramble an egg correctly anymore. Now it doesn't seem worth it to even go into the kitchen."

Sometimes during meals Susannah had trouble swallowing. If she did eat, she felt queasy for hours afterward. Her bowel movements were irregular, and her stomach upsets were keeping her awake at night.

"And I'm so jumpy, Dr. Vern," she said. "The slightest thing sets me off. I feel like a bundle of nerves."

Two Peas in a Pod

Patty and her husband Jake came to see me together. "It was this or a marriage counselor, and Patty doesn't look well, so we decided to start here," said Jake. "Patty says she can't stand her life anymore, and she wants to run away. But our kids need her. They love her. I love her. We are all worried about her."

As Jake spoke, Patty sat in the chair, looking at me with dull eyes. Her hair was unkempt, and her fingernails were chewed to the quick. "I just can't do this anymore," she said flatly. "Everyone expects so much of me, and I'm tired. I can't be a mother, a wife, a sex partner, a daughter, a sister, and a worker, and still be me. I used to be able to hold it all together. But something has changed. I know I should be able to keep doing all those things. But I just can't. I don't want to anymore. I guess I am a bad person. Something must be terribly wrong with me."

Who Is This Woman?

Many women who are experiencing stress feel like running away. It is a feeling that is alien to most women, especially because they are the ones who are usually most likely face problems head-on. That is why they have difficulty understanding their sudden desire to flee. Women under stress simply cannot deal with one more problem, question, or demand. This is just one of the many changes they don't understand.

This change in attitude is something their husbands don't understand, either. When I talk to husbands of women with female stress syndrome, they are baffled by the change that has taken place in their wives.

"She used to be so nice; nothing ever bothered her" is a common refrain from the husbands. "Now it seems that I can't do anything right. Neither can the kids."

Typically, the woman's response is something like, "I never used to feel this way.... This isn't me.... I'm not like this.... I don't like what I've become."

A Diary of Stress

Lori was a patient of mine about twelve years ago. She moved away and had three children and lived what she termed a "normally stressful life." Several more moves brought her back to Seattle and then again to see me for a sore ankle.

During my evaluation of Lori, she mentioned that she had periods of feeling achy all over and that a doctor had told her she might have fibromyalgia. As she continued, I began to understand that her ankle was only the tip of the iceberg. Unknowingly, she was describing many of the symptoms that relate to female stress syndrome. When I asked her if she felt she was under stress and that it was possible that her stress level was so intense that it could be the reason for her various conditions, she answered, "No," and quickly dismissed the notion as a long shot. I asked Lori to go home and write down what happened over the course of a typical day in her life and bring it when she returned for her follow-up visit for her ankle. This is what she wrote:

Lately I feel like I'm aging quickly every day. In the past five years I feel that I've become too serious about everyday life. My life has become a chore. Whether it be my personality or something in my past, I feel the need to meet some kind of criteria. In the process I've lost my way. I have forgotten the meaning of life, and I have lost my youth.

I have a lot to be thankful for. I have three beautiful children, a wonderful husband, and everything I could ever need or want. Still, I have so many things to do to keep this household running. I must keep everyone happy and healthy, and keep up with sports and school. So many days I feel like a robot. No smiling, no laughing, just drudge through until the kids go to bed, which is my chance to sit and do nothing. Yet my mind keeps going. The schedule for the whole week is going through my mind; don't forget this, remember that. I fall asleep on the couch and wake up a half-hour later with an anxiety attack.

What is wrong with me? I go to bed and think. Most nights I'm in some kind of state between sleep and wakefulness. I sometimes have terrible hallucinations that there are demons, devils, or witches in my room and that my husband is some *thing* other than himself, and of course I wake up in a panic. Then I'm restless all night only to wake up at 5:30 A.M. to my husband's wonderful kiss goodbye. Then my eight-year-old crawls in at 6:30 A.M.; my four-year-old at 7:00 A.M., and my two-year-old cries out at 7:30 A.M.

So I go to bed tired and wake up feeling like a Mack truck ran over me. Now I'm cranky while trying to organize the morning on no sleep. Already starting to raise my voice to get everyone ready for school. Some days I wake up and say, "Today will be the day I relax and do nothing," but that has never happened. A cup of coffee gives me my second wind, and I'm off cleaning and cooking, driving to school, carpooling, gymnastics, health club, etc. . . . etc. . . . while thinking, "Have I smiled today?"

There's so much to do that there's no time for fun or laughter. Go, go, go. Then by 3:00 P.M. I'm exhausted, and it's time for school to let out. My oldest daughter comes home and I'm in the same mood as when she left. Time for dinner and soccer and baths. Then the guilt sets in. I'm missing out on my daughter's life. Where is the fun and love and play? I'm a terrible mother because I don't pull myself away from tasks to enjoy my children. Taking care of them and my home is a job. I do enjoy them now and again, but I know I will have plenty of regrets later when it's all gone.

I feel at least three times a week that I must be going insane. I try to keep myself together. I'm the operator of this house, so if anything goes wrong, it must be my fault. I blame myself for any problems, that may arise during the week. I want to run away . . . but run away to what? I really want to make changes, but I think I need some healing. How can I listen to my children and help them emotionally when I am an emotional wreck?

I stress out over silly things and can't cope. I have told myself many times that knowing the problem is halfway to solving, so I'll solve it. But I'm starting to realize there is something wrong. No sleep, night sweats, chest pains, numbness in my chest, headaches, knee pain, elbow pain, neck pain, feeling light-headed, getting optic migraines; the list goes on and on. The more pain I feel the more anxious I get. Sometimes I feel I can't cope outside of this life that I've made for myself. I really want to change things, but the thought of change makes me very nervous. On top of all that, I feel the need to look great and stay healthy; I'm worried about what people think. Will I ever find peace?

As you read through this book, you will come to understand how you, like Lori, may have become highly stressed. You will find that you are not alone in the experiences and behaviors that are occurring in your life, and that they are more predictable than you may have realized.

In the next chapter you will see that hormone imbalances play a major role in driving your behavior and causing these unpleasant and distressing symptoms. Understanding the cause of your problems is the first step toward learning how to take the necessary steps to regain control of your life.

CHAPTER TWO

Biology Drives Behavior

Chronic stress and its accompanying health woes begin with a normal reaction commonly known as the fight-or-flight response. Millions of years of evolution have endowed us with the means to fight or flee a host of potential threats. Our prehistoric ancestors, whether hunting or being hunted, needed quick jolts of energy to run faster, hit harder, and see and hear better. When confronted by a threat such as a hungry tiger, their brains set in motion a response that supercharged their bodies with energy and shut down all functions not needed for the immediate struggle.

The fight-or-flight response is controlled in our bodies by a system called the sympathetic nervous system. Alongside this system is the feed-or-breed system, known to doctors as the parasympathetic nervous system. Both of these systems are controlled by the brain and are influenced by events and experiences that we encounter. When we are faced with danger the sympathetic system prepares us for battle or to run away—fast! Simultaneously, it shuts down parasympathetic functions such as eating, digesting, and breeding, that is, sexuality. Our fight-or-flight response was designed for the *occasional* episode of sudden threat—the tiger leaping into our path. It was *not* designed to be engaged throughout a 24-hours-a-day, seven-days-a-week life of chaos, overscheduling, and excessive stress. When our nervous system goes into overdrive, the result is overproduction of our "warrior hormones" and underproduction of other hormones, like DHEA, critical to our health and happiness.

Today, although we generally don't encounter tigers or similar threats on a daily basis, our bodies still respond to acute stress in the same manner as they did millennia ago. Everything from falling in love to speaking before an audience can precipitate a fight-or-flight response. To some, the tiger would be a lesser threat!

When Your Brain Senses Stress

The biological response to stress begins in your brain. As stated earlier, when your brain perceives a stressor, your sympathetic nervous system, which controls and fuels the fight-or-flight response, kicks into action.

First, a small area in your brain (about the size of the tip of your thumb) called the hypothalamus sends a message to the adrenal glands. The two adrenal glands, or adrenals, each sits atop the kidney, right in the middle of the body. When you are stressed, the adrenal glands quickly flood your body with adrenaline and noradrenaline. These chemicals instantly send your blood pressure soaring and cause your heart to pump faster, increasing blood flow to meet its high demand. Your skin might feel cool during stress as blood is diverted from it to more essential organs that allow you to respond to the perceived threat. Your stomach may feel tight for the same reason. Blood is being diverted from the digestive system and away from the sexual organs. Adrenaline and noradrenaline also quicken your breathing and dilate your eyes to let in more light. When they reach your brain, adrenaline and noradrenaline trigger an emotional response to the stress and suppress short-term memory, concentration, inhibition, and rational thought. You can think and act quickly, but you won't be able to handle complex intellectual tasks because your animal responses will dominate your rational ones. This response is the reason we may say or do things in times of panic or stress that we later regret. It is also the reason why we can perform tasks never thought possible, with increased and unusual strength, when the threat is severe enough.

Master Control

The hypothalamus is the key control center for the regulation of growth, sex, and reproduction, in addition to intense emotions like fear, rage, and ecstatic pleasure. It is the master controller of a complex sequence of events that occur in each and every person confronted with the varied experiences that can be characterized as threatening. The hypothalamus exerts powerful control and influence over the body and does not respond to well-intentioned, rational urgings to be calm. In my own personal experience, I have noticed that my naive attempts to calm a woman under significant hypothalamic influence by advising her to "just settle down" are tantamount to throwing gasoline on a raging fire. Fortunately, in the clinical arena I have become more proficient at helping women understand what is happening to them, biologically, when they feel as though they are going to explode, and helping them find more effective means of managing these sensations.

When you experience unrestrained, high levels of hypothalamus stress stimulation, an intense signal is sent throughout the body via adrenaline. Without DHEA, estrogen, progesterone, or testosterone to offset or oppose it, panic can set in. The muscles begin to tighten and prepare for action. As the chest wall expands to fill with oxygen, breathing deepens and accelerates to circulate high levels of this needed fuel to muscle cells. The heart beats faster and harder, often causing the feeling that it is beating outside the chest. Blood vessels are constricted, or narrowed, by the stress hormone surge, and blood pressure rises quickly. The vasoconstriction can be so intense that the skin can literally turn white from lack of blood flow. The abundance of unopposed adrenaline can cause sweating, tachycardia (fast heart rate), throbbing headaches, chest pressure, chest pain, feelings of impending doom, shortness of breath, trembling or shaking, dry mouth, and insomnia.

The Biological Source of Panic

It is estimated that upward of 10% of the population now suffer from social phobia syndrome and panic attacks. These anxiety states are largely caused by heightened and sustained levels of adrenaline and other stress-induced biological mechanisms, resulting in a continued state of panic without the ability, or "biology," to counteract this high-energy body state.

During stress, the adrenal glands also release cortisol, a chemical so integral to stress it is often called the stress hormone. Cortisol is a warrior hormone and is secreted in abundance when we are in a constant state of threat.

Your cortisol levels vary throughout the day during normal living. Higher levels typically occur in the mornings and tend to taper off during the night. Your brain monitors signals from the body and can turn up or turn down the production of cortisol as needed.

Cortisol fuels your stressed body with glucose, a sugar. Glucose is an energy source for your body. Initially, the liver releases its reserves of glucose stores in response to stress. It then begins to break down and convert proteins in your body to glucose. With all that sugar flowing through your blood, your body is primed for physical action. Cortisol also suppresses parts of your immune system and reduces any inflammation that might result if tissue is damaged during the fighting or fleeing.

During this time of responding to threat, once cortisol levels surge, we try our best to adapt to the situation. Dr. Hans Selye, an endocrinologist recognized as the father of stress studies, demonstrated that we pass through three phases during what is called the adaptation response to a stressful situation. The alarm phase of adaptation encompasses the bodily changes described above. The second phase in the stress response is a resistance stage, when the revved-up body processes drift back to normal. Even in the presence of the continued stress, we accommodate to it and biological parameters such as blood pressure and pulse return to normal levels. In the last phase, called exhaustion, the alarmlike reactions reappear. Blood pressure and pulse again increase, as do other processes, such as deeper breathing. Unfortunately, it is difficult for the body to regain control of this situation, and significant irreparable damage to the body's internal organs can occur.

Fight, Run, or Hide?

The way we deal with the ebb and flow of stresses in our lives is critically dependent on the biological balancing of the various hormones involved in our body's response to stress. Some interesting behaviors are seen in people suffering from continued unrelenting stress. These behaviors, largely determined by the biological state of the person at the time, are both common and predictable.

For many people under a mild amount of daily stress, their learned behaviors can balance the incoming levels of stress. They may increase their exercise to compensate for the day's added stress or get a massage.

They may talk to an empathetic friend or work in the garden, read, or listen to music. All these behaviors, or coping techniques, are considered good, well-balanced attempts at pushing back against the stress encountered that day.

Others, as stress increases to the point of near overload, find themselves feeling more and more anxious, apprehensive, and fearful. They rapidly begin to increase their level of activity, as if preparing for an impending storm. They begin searching for solutions to their current dilemma, trying to find money to pay the bills or time to complete overdue tasks. This increased pressure can sometimes make people very creative. As an example, when my colleagues and I were faced with ever-increasing deficits due to the negative impact of managed care in our state, we were forced to formulate new ideas to survive the situation. As we mulled over the stressful reality of losing money every month in our otherwise very busy practices, we created a logical solution. We would not have been this creative unless we were thrust into a perilous situation, causing us to expand our abilities to seek out viable answers to solve our problem. Many important discoveries, artistic achievements, and business innovations come from people confronted with stresses that they choose to overcome.

Overload—that feeling of the wave crashing on top of you, of feeling buried, overwhelmed, with no end or solution in sight—can cause you to feel crushed by the weight of your burdens. We may not be able to compensate effectively for the feeling of having more to do than can possibly be done. This is when other predictable coping behaviors begin to show. As you are continually consumed by more than you can handle, that feeling of the room closing in on you worsens. Some of us begin to crumble, unable to handle anything more than basic everyday tasks. For others, even these simple chores are too much. These people decompensate, deflate, become more sedentary, and expend less and less effort as the feeling of discouragement increases. Exhaustion sets in along with increased depression and feelings of poor self-esteem.

Personality comes into play during periods of sustained and intense stress. Core values and deeply ingrained learned behaviors will show themselves as people retreat to their basic nature. Some individuals become more cautious than usual and take fewer risks during this time, if that is their basic nature. Others simply run away, leaving all the "badness" behind them to try to begin a new life, elsewhere. Some people retreat and avoid the situation as best they can, denying (or trying to) that the problem exists. Like an ostrich, they survive by putting their head in the sand and hoping the problems will just go away. A person who drinks alcohol to relax and escape will increase this coping behavior. Smokers will smoke more; eaters will consume more food; gamblers will increase their bets. All of these behaviors, though self-destructive, are the best such people can do for themselves without outside intervention.

Understanding the biological impact of stress and using the various tools and techniques discussed in this book can help you avoid the trap of a self-destructive stress response and give you new opportunities to rise above the situation and prosper.

Performance and Stress

Under periods of intense and persistent stress, people simply perform more poorly. They have less ability to tolerate the gray areas of life and become more black and white in their thinking. They have a decreased ability to make even simple decisions. They make more mistakes and have a harder time prioritizing.

During these periods of high stress and poor performance, your life environment is an important factor in your ability to improve the stressful situation or worsen it. A study at the University of Maryland revealed that when given supportive comments and reassurance during these periods of ineffective behavior, people tended to improve their performance and lessen their destructive behaviors. Conversely, when more pressure was added, such as increased verbal accusations and threats regarding poor performance, people decompensated further and their poor coping behaviors increased. Both situations—extremely high stress over a short period or moderately high stress for an extended period—can cause the behaviors discussed above and the resulting decompensation.

The worst scenario is extremely high stress that occurs over long periods of time. This situation is increasingly becoming a reality for many of my patients and others across the country. As evidenced by laboratory analysis of over 2,500 patients, the biological response to stress is evident. Women and men alike are consuming their stress-coping hormones, such as DHEA, faster than they can produce them. The result is a decreased ability to cope with daily life, behaviors unbecoming to the person, and frustration with the medical profession due to its ongoing lack of answers and effective solutions.

DHEA: The Balancing Hormone

DHEA has been called a hormone precursor, or prohormone, because it is ultimately converted into the sex hormones: testosterone, progesterone, and estrogen. But make no mistake: Precursor or not, DHEA is an active substance that exerts a powerful influence over your body functions.

DHEA is manufactured primarily by the adrenal glands, but it is also made by the testicles, ovaries, and the brain. Over the last several years research on DHEA has been increasing at a phenomenal rate. As researchers have begun to evaluate the direct effects of DHEA, they have discovered that this prohormone is not just a stepping-stone to other bioactive molecules. DHEA itself is a rather large "stone" that can be thrown at our stresses to improve our ability to cope with them.

DHEA appears to be a buffering hormone, offsetting the effects of the other stress-related hormones we've discussed. I call DHEA "the coping fuel" and "the universal promoter of goodness" due to its effects as a balancing hormone. If cortisol is the hormone we call on to battle the various wars of life, DHEA is the hormone that offsets cortisol. (To discuss the complex interplay of these biological opponents within the scope of this book, I have had to simplify the discussion of their actual biochemical activities. In an effort not to dilute the science, however, I refer the scientific community and interested readers to the reference section for a more detailed description of these biochemical interactions.)

Cortisol and DHEA work as opposites. During a period of stress, cortisol has a tearing-down effect on the body, breaking proteins into glucose in an effort to fight the fight. Once the stressful situation passes, cortisol production is shut off and DHEA is produced to restore calm and balance. When the stress becomes chronic, nearly all of your nutritional resources are sent to your adrenal glands so that they will continue to produce cortisol. This preferential production of cortisol shortchanges the production of DHEA, making your body unable to maintain the levels of DHEA required for peak performance. As your DHEA levels diminish and you remain in a state of hypervigilance, you cannot muster the fuel to cope with the continual threats cast upon you.

Why Are We Still Fighting Tigers?

Even though we no longer live unprotected in the wild, you still need your body's stress response. Some stress is a necessary ingredient in your life, and the fight-or-flight response is still a valuable defense mechanism. It may give you the energy to meet a demanding deadline or make a quick decision in a crisis.

Take the case of Bonnie, a petite dynamo. Bonnie has had to endure more than life's usual hardships. She put her husband through school while taking care of her two young daughters. He filed for divorce soon after he graduated. To support herself, she went to school at night and worked by day. Like most single mothers, Bonnie was experiencing an overwhelming amount of chronic stress.

Finally, Bonnie met a young man with whom she had so many common interests that they eventually moved in together to give family life a try. Things went well for several months until one day a trivial argument turned explosive. Before Bonnie knew it, her boyfriend was screaming at the top of his lungs and lunged at her. "He completely lost control. He had never done this before and had no history of this kind of behavior. He just snapped," she said.

Bonnie's fight-or-flight response kicked in immediately. She threw her boyfriend to the floor and ran to a phone to call the police.

Bonnie's display of Herculean strength and warriorlike response was not planned or plotted. It happened instantly; it was pure reaction. This is how the fight-or-flight response works. We don't have time to think, "I'd better transfer some glucose from my liver to my bloodstream now and dilate my arteries to increase blood flow to my muscles." The process happens with laserlike precision and is very effective at allowing us to either stay and fight or run away in flight.

Normally, a stress reaction fades as soon as the body restores calm or once a threat is gone. As the warrior hormones recede, calming biological molecules are released to calm the storm. The parasympathetic nervous system takes over, fostering the feed-or-breed response. Assuming you have an adequate supply of these counteractive biochemical messengers, your heart rate and blood flow return to normal, and your sex drive and appetite return. If continued stress has inhibited or exhausted your body's ability to produce these important hormones, however, your return to normal will be compromised.

When Stress Turns Bad

Your body can usually tell the difference between real threats and life's minor annoyances and frustrations, such as long lines at the store, traffic jams, or even normal, everyday arguments. But sometimes your fight-or-flight mechanism gets stuck in the on position, when every threat seems to bring on the fight response, and you feel as though you have a simmering kettle of nerves under the surface just waiting to boil over. Your body continues to pump out cortisol in response to the constant pressures of daily life. Over time all this cortisol has a negative effect on other important hormones that normally keep one another in check. Your body was not designed to be under the influence of these warrior hormones day in and day out. Sustained and prolonged elevation of adrenaline and cortisol begins to take a major toll on the stability of the body's psychological and physiological buffering systems.

The Age Factor

When we are young our DHEA levels climb steadily. DHEA reaches maximum level at about age 25. After age 30 DHEA begins to decline slowly. That decline continues as we age. By age 90 DHEA has dropped to 10% of its maximum level.

As women enter premenopause (in their 30s), perimenopause (in their 40s), or menopause (in their 50s), the effects of low DHEA become much more pronounced. With menopause a woman's ovaries begin to lose function, and with that loss of function follows a drop in estrogen. Progesterone and testosterone are also declining during this time. Among other things, estrogen and progesterone are critically involved in a woman's ability to cope effectively with day-to-day stress. With the decline in DHEA, estrogen, progesterone, and testosterone, a woman has fewer hormonal resources to balance her emotions and cope with stress.

The decline in DHEA levels is now occurring at a much earlier age, at a much faster rate, and to much lower levels than ever before. Today DHEA levels approach their peak in a woman's midtwenties rather than in her thirties, and begin to drop rapidly after this time. This means that DHEA is dropping to critically low levels much earlier than what would be considered normal.

This rapid decline is coupled with an increased inability to cope with even the slightest of life's provocations. I believe this phenomenon is a direct result of excessive stress caused by increasingly demanding lifestyles overwhelming the body's ability to produce essential coping hormones, such as DHEA.

DHEA Affects Other Hormones

When persistent stress and prolonged levels of increased cortisol deplete DHEA, they also reduce other key hormones such as estrogen, progesterone, and testosterone.

Diminished or fluctuating levels of estrogen and progesterone can cause irritability, anger, frustration, tearfulness, depression, and a wide range of emotions associated with the female stress syndrome. Since estrogen and testosterone are key to bone formation and maturation, when levels of these hormones fall bone density can decline, making a woman a prime target for osteoporosis.

While testosterone is commonly known as a male hormone, it is also a key "hormone of desire" for many women. Many female patients suffer from a lack of libido and have a difficult time achieving sexual satisfaction when stress levels are consistently high. Testosterone is also responsible for proper glucose regulation. Low levels of testosterone can lead to obesity and diabetes, a decrease in muscle tone and muscle mass, and a decrease in bone density, which may progress to osteoporosis. DHEA acts as a precursor, or building block, for helping testosterone levels return to a normal and healthy level.

The Not-So-Normal Thyroid

Thyroid hormone, too, can be disrupted by too much stress over a long period. Under normal circumstances the brain signals the thyroid gland to secrete its hormone in the inactive, or storage, form called T_4. The T_4 hormone is then activated outside the thyroid gland in the body's tissues and converted to T_3, which elevates metabolism. Several biological mechanisms must be in place for this occur.

When everything is working correctly, the basal body temperature remains close to the normal 98.6 degrees. When stress-related disruptions occur in this process, thyroid hormone begins to decrease in effectiveness.

To conserve energy the body converts less T_4 to T_3 and more T_4 to Reverse T_3 (RT_3), another less active form. RT_3 actually blocks T_3 from working normally. This causes the body to function at a slower pace, which patients experience as fatigue. Physicians frequently fail to notice decreased thyroid functioning, despite patient complaints of fatigue and weight gain—both hallmarks of impaired thyroid functioning—because traditional tests appear normal. Health care providers are also very resistant to pursuing this thyroid dysfunction further because their traditional training did not teach them anything about this type of thyroid abnormality. Unfortunately, many physicians hold the opinion that if they haven't learned something it must not be valid or true.

It appears, however, that some doctors are beginning to learn and understand new areas of medicine that are based more in functionality and nutritional biochemistry, opening more doors for patients to be treated effectively. The debate over thyroid dysfunction, in the context of "normal" thyroid laboratory values, is a prime example of this trend. I have treated many patients with small amounts of T_3 along with DHEA supplementation, reversing the "blockage" of producing T_3 normally. Fatigue abates, other bodily functions return to normal, and the constellations of other symptoms that accompany this abnormal thyroid phenomenon are rapidly diminished.

In addition to thyroid function returning to normal, progesterone and other DHEA-derived female hormones begin to return to normal levels as DHEA stores are replenished. Improved hormone levels go a long way to reverse the ongoing emotional and physical trauma caused by excessive stress. The body can begin to correct itself with proper nourishment, including increased intake of certain nutritional supplements. Targeted nutrition combined with a better perspective of why your behavior is the way it is allows you to understand more completely what is happening to you and what you can do about it. In my community seminars about female stress syndrome, I spend a significant amount of time explaining how biology drives behavior, which we've reviewed in this chapter. This concept may allow you not only to understand how you tick, but also why others around you behave as they do when under stress.

Women Are the Most Affected

Evidence is emerging that the stressed state might be more pronounced in women than in men. Studies by the National Institute of Child Health and

Human Development and the University of Michigan found that estrogen may increase cortisol secretion and decrease the ability of cortisol to shut down its own secretion. The result might be a stress response that is not only more pronounced but also longer-lasting in women than in men.

Stress and Disease

Over time a constant state of stress causes wear and tear on your body. This is not just psychologically unpleasant, it is also physically damaging. The most obvious effects are tension headaches, anxiety, sore muscles, exhaustion, and insomnia. But researchers also link chronic stress to a variety of more serious health problems.

Since DHEA is used by nearly every tissue of the body for proper functioning, it stands to reason that as DHEA levels decline there is a decrease in the body's ability to remain healthy that can lead to serious illness. The longer the stress to the body, the more damage done to its vital systems. In fact, a lack of DHEA is related to almost every major disease, from diabetes, cardiovascular disease, and immune disorders to depression and other mental disease, osteoporosis, and even cancer.

In 1990 Mohammed Kalimi, Ph.D., and William Regelson, M.D., brought together the latest information at the time relating to DHEA research. Their book, *The Biological Role of Dehydroepiandrosterone (DHEA)*, presented scientific evidence from all corners of the world and gave the following overview of the benefit of DHEA: "DHEA modulates diabetes, obesity, carcinogenesis, tumor growth, neurite outgrowth, virus and bacterial infection, stress, pregnancy, hypertension, collagen and skin integrity, fatigue, depression, memory, and immune responses." The evidence at the time supported the prohormone role of DHEA and focused on its effects as a precursor hormone leading to a "host of steroid progeny." There is no doubt that the effects of DHEA are far-reaching and are very influential in the body's ability to maintain a healthy level of functioning.

Diabetes

Constant stress messages being sent to the adrenal glands cause excess glucose to be maintained in the bloodstream. Increased glucose stimulates the pancreas to release and maintain elevated levels of circulating insulin in the bloodstream to "escort" glucose into cells for energy and return blood glucose levels to normal. Low DHEA, combined with other nutritional deficiencies—such as chromium deficiency, for instance—leads to insulin resistance, in which elevated insulin levels circulate in the bloodstream but are ineffective in controlling and bringing blood sugar to optimal levels. Insulin resistance is a key risk factor for weight gain and type 2 diabetes.

DHEA also inhibits the effects an enzyme called G6PD (glucose-6-phosphate dehydrogenase), which is partly responsible for fat storage. This is why DHEA supplementation can lead to weight loss. Studies have shown that DHEA may improve glucose usage, a key component in the prevention or correction of diabetes. Findings published in the *International Journal of Obesity* in 1986 noted the antiobesity effects of DHEA, along with a decrease in the severity of diabetes.

In addition, DHEA has been shown to decrease elevated levels of insulin. Volunteers who took 100 mg of DHEA for 30 days decreased their insulin levels by 27%. Conversely, in 1997 a study published in the journal *Metabolism* showed that insulin resistance resulting in higher levels of circulating insulin actually decreased DHEA levels in the blood. The study also showed that DHEA levels were inversely related to body fat, meaning that increased DHEA levels were associated with less fat and more muscle, and lower DHEA levels were associated with increased body fat.

Cardiovascular Disease

A review of studies at the Medical College of Wisconsin revealed that the repeated blood pressure elevations caused by chronic stress may eventually lead to chronic hypertension. Other studies show that people with the highest stress levels are roughly twice as likely to have high blood pressure as individuals under normal stress. This stress-related health problem can have serious consequences. Over time stress-induced increases in blood pressure may cause your arteries to become thicker and less elastic, which can lead to atherosclerosis, in which fatty material accumulates under the inner lining of your arterial walls. When atherosclerosis develops in the arteries that supply the heart, a heart attack may occur. Blockage and damage to the carotid arteries (the arteries that supply blood to your brain) are the primary causes of stroke.

In a 1986 study published in the *New England Journal of Medicine*, Elizabeth Barrett-Conner, M.D., highlighted the positive cardiovascular effects of DHEA. Working in the Department of Family Medicine at the University of California School of Medicine in San Diego, she followed DHEA levels in 242 men aged 50–79 for 12 years. She found that an increase in DHEA by 100 mcg/dl (micrograms per deciliter) resulted in a decreased mortality (death rate) of 36% from any cause. She found that the death rate from cardiovascular disease decreased by 48% with only a modest 100-point increase in DHEA.

A good deal of research has focused on the link between emotional stress and heart disease. For example, a recent study of nearly 1,000 middle-aged Finnish citizens found that arteries narrowed more quickly in those who reported high levels of hopelessness than in those who were more optimistic about the future. Another study of more than 7,000 British government workers found that, after an average of five years, clerks and office staff were more likely to develop coronary heart disease than those in higher-grade jobs. The authors suggest that simple, monotonous work over which one has little control is more stressful than a demanding job over which one has some influence. A feeling of lack of control leads to anger and frustration, which can lead to high blood pressure, which can then lead to heart disease. Numerous other studies have reported that angry, hostile people are more likely to suffer a heart attack than people who are more relaxed.

The fight-or-flight response also causes blood to become stickier. This may help to prepare your body for immediate blood clotting should an injury occur. Research shows that stress increases the rate of clot and plaque formation even when other factors, such as diet, remain unchanged. This action increases the likelihood of blood clots in the arteries around the heart.

In 1995 Robert L. Jesse, M.D., published a paper in the *Annals of the New York Academy of Sciences* showing that DHEA decreases the stickiness of platelets. That effect of DHEA decreases the chance of blood clotting leading to heart attack or stroke. Other research has shown that even 50 mg per day of DHEA for 12 days improved the ability of patients to dissolve fibrin in blood clots.

Stress may also signal the body to release fat into the bloodstream, raising blood cholesterol levels. In women stress may reduce estrogen levels, which are important and protective for heart health.

Even periods of mild stress were found to increase levels of homocysteine, an amino acid associated with heart disease. An Ohio State University study of 34 middle-aged women found that even brief periods of stress increased levels of the substance, which is a serious risk factor in heart disease. Homocysteine, a metabolite of protein breakdown, is a potent promoter of the process of hardening of the arteries known as atherosclerosis.

Immune Disorders

When activated by the fight-or-flight response, cortisol suppresses your immune system by decreasing the production of lymphocytes (especially T cells) and antibodies. DHEA promotes a generalized immune response and counteracts the immuno-suppressing effects of corticosteroids like cortisol. With chronic stress, cortisol runs rampant and DHEA production cannot keep pace offsetting its effects. Several studies have verified that subjects under chronic stress have low white blood cell counts and are more vulnerable to colds, infections, and allergies. People feeling overwhelmed by life events have been shown to have one-third the normal levels of natural killer (NK) cells in their body. DHEA also converts to other, even more active metabolites that promote immunity. It is important to note that DHEA itself is not directly responsible for the increased immunity. DHEA confers its benefits by enhancing the activity of lymphocytes, lymphoid organs, and other immune hormones called cytokines.

Women who are highly stressed may be at increased risk for vaginal infections due to candida (yeast). Many of my patients report that as soon as they get over one yeast infection they find that they have developed another. This can also cause tension in the bedroom, as yeast irritates the vaginal mucosa and can make sexual intimacy very painful. Each less-than-fulfilling sexual experience only adds more stress to the equation. Usually a few days of a topical antifungal medication are all that is needed to alleviate this problem. I rarely have to prescribe oral medication. In fact, many of my patients have had their symptoms disappear once their DHEA levels have been restored to normal.

Stress can reduce your immunity to all sorts of diseases. Alice, a 40-year-old special events manager, was recently put in charge of the most important project of her life: a major international meeting. As the event date drew near, Alice began putting in ever-increasing hours at work to fulfill her obligations. Ultimately, she found herself working 16-hour days. Of course, sleep, nutrition, and most other aspects of her life fell by the wayside. Finally this exhausting schedule culminated in the "event of a lifetime." The two weeks of the event itself seemed like one long day to her.

"I just went from fire to fire and problem to problem for about two weeks, nonstop," she said. "After it was over, I just collapsed."

But Alice had not come to see me about stress. She came to ask me about the intense pain and the blisters that had broken out over her forehead. Alice had a case of shingles (herpes zoster). This is very unusual for someone her age. Shingles is more typically seen in patients aged 65–70.

I told Alice that her frenetic way of life had turned into a war on her body and that now she was shell-shocked—literally. Because the shingles was so close to her eyes, I referred her to an ophthalmologist for immediate treatment with high-dose antiviral medications and potent anti-inflammatory medications. By the time of her two-week follow-up visit, Alice was almost fully recovered.

As it turned out, on the same day that Alice came in for her checkup, another of my patients was diagnosed with shingles, though not as severe. The unusual point again was her age: She was only 38 years old! She had recently taken a corporate job, only to realize that her personality did not fit corporate life—or her new position. Ultimately, she ended up quitting after only two weeks. In addition to the unusual herpes zoster outbreak, she had daily diarrhea, cramps, muscle tension, headaches, and a severe outbreak of dermatitis. She was able to return to her old job but with a new perspective. She was much happier, and within a few days her symptoms began to go away.

I had never before seen two cases of stress-induced shingles in the same day, let alone in such young patients. My approach to both of them was to point out that their severe levels of stress and personal neglect invited the herpes zoster virus into their bodies and let it "set up shop" and begin taking its devastating toll. Manifestations of the herpes virus (HV), whether as a cold sore, genital herpes, or shingles, are all associated with major stressful events. I put both patients on DHEA and major stress reduction programs.

Depression

Stress is also almost invariably linked to depression, which is twice as common in women as men. Studies have found that approximately half of all patients with major depression have high levels of cortisol. But is stress a symptom or a cause of depression? Most researchers believe that it is a two-way street: Stress affects depression, and depression affects stress.

Recent research suggests that high cortisol levels are one possible cause of depression. Researchers at the University of California in San Francisco believe that stress hormones influence serotonin, dopamine, and other neurotransmitters in the brain. Imbalances in the biochemistry of the brain and a shortage of serotonin and/or dopamine (or a relative imbalance between serotonin and dopamine) are related to depression.

The fact that women are more prone to depression than men might also be rooted in the relationship between cortisol and estrogen. As mentioned earlier, research has shown that during stressful events estrogen not only increases cortisol secretion, but also decreases the ability of cortisol to shut down its own secretion. A study at the University of Michigan showed that women have longer-lasting cortisol responses during the high-estrogen phase of their menstrual cycles. Researchers believe that this relationship may explain why women are more prone to depression, especially after a stressful event.

Other Mental Effects

Studies show that high levels of cortisol interfere with memory. A study at the Washington University School of Medicine exposed subjects to high cortisol levels for several days. These were the same levels that might occur with a major physical or psychological stressor. Subjects experienced memory impairment after four days of high cortisol. When their cortisol levels dropped, their memory performance returned to normal. Other studies suggest that if stress is chronic or extremely severe, memory loss may become permanent. Researchers believe that cortisol interferes with the energy supply to certain brain cells involved in memory.

Bone Loss

A study in Germany linked depression with bone loss, and again the connection was high cortisol levels. Cortisol increases bone resorption (the bone proteins are converted to quick energy) and decreases bone formation by inhibiting calcium absorption. Over time more of your bone mass is reabsorbed and less is rebuilt because less calcium is taken up. The result is osteopenia (moderate bone loss and weakening) or osteoporosis (major bone loss and weakening) in both men and women. DHEA has been positively associated with vertebral bone density in postmenopausal women and is likely a protective factor against osteoporosis.

A study in Japan of 120 postmenopausal women documented a positive relationship between DHEA and bone mineral density. DHEA is thought to regulate bone density by affecting osteoclasts (bone-absorbing cells) as well as osteoblasts (bone-forming cells). Cytokines, chemical messengers similar to hormones that affect immunity and can be inflammatory-causing agents, can generate "free radicals," which activate osteoclasts, the cells that cause bone absorption and lead to weaker bone structure. As people grow older, their levels of pro-inflammatory cytokines increase, which in turn increases the production of free radicals. Research shows that DHEA reverses the increase of several pro-inflammatory cytokines that occurs naturally with age.

Cancer

Researchers are exploring the link between stress and serious diseases like cancer. A Stanford University School of Medicine study tracked women with terminal breast cancer and found that those with abnormally high levels of cortisol were significantly more likely to die sooner than women with lower levels of cortisol. An earlier study at Stanford found that women with advanced breast cancer who participated in programs offering emotional support and training lived twice as long as those who did not participate. This finding does not mean that stress causes cancer, but this and other studies support the belief that emotional states influence the progression or regression of disease.

Research studies from England reported in 1971 indicated that low levels of DHEA were associated with breast cancer. The study found that the risk was increased even if women had low levels up to nine years prior to the diagnosis. In 1979, Arthur Schwartz, M.D., of Temple University reported in *Cancer Research* that long-term treatment with DHEA inhibited spontaneous breast cancer formation in female mice. He indicated that DHEA protected cells from the toxicity of carcinogens. Dr. Schwartz's research was focused on the protective effect that DHEA provides to cells. When cells are confronted with carcinogenic agents, they undergo mutations or changes in their DNA, transformations or changes in form or appearance, and increased cell death. Schwartz found that when DHEA was added to the carcinogenic material, the cells showed much less effect from the cancer-causing agents.

Sexual and Reproductive Function

Stress can lead to intensified premenstrual syndrome (PMS), diminished sexual desire, and irregular menstruation. In cases of severely elevated cortisol, menstruation may shut down altogether.

A Danish study showed that women under high levels of stress who also have a longer than average menstrual cycle have a decreased fertility rate and an increased miscarriage rate. Stress during pregnancy has been linked to a 50% higher risk of miscarriage, as well as lower birth weights and premature births. The stress response may interfere with normal blood flow to the placenta.

I practiced obstetrics for the first several years of my practice, and in my experience it was not uncommon for a woman to have a spontaneous miscarriage following a major stressful event in her life. The stress of an unplanned pregnancy can also be too much, emotionally, for some patients. When that happens, their internal mechanisms take over and "decide" that the time is not right for the body to mature the fetus, ending in a miscarriage. I also have seen increased stress put patients into premature labor as the body fights to prioritize its allocation of resources under adverse conditions. For those trying to become pregnant, stress can make conception unattainable until the level of stress is diminished.

Stress and the Hormone Roller Coaster

To fully understand how stress interferes with pregnancy we must first understand the normal female hormonal system. As we have learned earlier, the hypothalamus is the main regulatory gland in the brain that controls mood, libido, thirst, appetite, sleep, body temperature, and blood pressure. Every month the hypothalamus normally releases a special hormone targeted to reproduction called gonadotropin-releasing hormone (GnRH). Its chemical message is received by the pituitary gland, another small yet powerful master gland that lies deep in the brain, just above the sinuses. This chemical signal tells the pituitary to release two other hormones, follicle-stimulating hormone (FSH) and luteinizing hormone (LH). These two hormones target the ovaries, stimulating them to prepare for ovulation.

This process can be greatly affected by our emotional state. GnRH is affected by other familiar brain chemicals such as norepinehrine (which speeds up its release) and serotonin and dopamine (which inhibit it). As these brain chemicals change in response to the increased or decreased stresses in our lives, so does the menstrual cycle. Once the sequence becomes totally disrupted, ovulation can be interrupted or anovulation can occur, stopping ovulation completely.

A second hormonal problem involves prolactin levels. Prolactin is a natural birth control hormone that the body produces, especially in breast-feeding mothers, following a pregnancy. It inhibits the secretion of FSH, so follicles do not mature and ovulation does not occur. Studies have shown that prolactin levels are high in times of acute or chronic stress. Thus, women with high stress levels often have irregular cycles or no ovulation at all.

The third problem deals with the so-called stress hormones. When stress occurs at an increased frequency or at sustained levels, the body's fight-or-flight response takes over and the hormones adrenaline and noradrenaline are released. This interferes with the release of gonadotropin-releasing hormone, GnRH, changing or inhibiting the ovulation cycle. Women can experience up to 50 brief fight-or-flight episodes each day! Whether these are as threatening as an attempt on our lives, or as innocuous as the alarm going off in the morning, our bodies respond in the same way. Once the adrenaline is released, it takes hours to dissipate. So, if you are subjected to many stressful moments in your day, your menstrual cycle could be severely disrupted.

Stress and Infertility

Many couples who suffer from infertility undergo incredible amounts of stress when they seek professional treatment to conquer this problem. Many infertility treatments are expensive, painful, and involve tense waiting periods living under a microscope, literally and figuratively. Women may begin to feel depressed and not in control of their lives, leading to more stress, which may complicate treatment and threaten a positive outcome.

Madison and Greg illustrate the stress associated with trying to get pregnant. Madison is a hard-driving professional, always going beyond what is asked of her and always in demand by those at her work. She knew all the answers and ran circles around the men at the financial consulting business where she spent most of her long days. Madison's working 60 hours a week, taking aerobics classes, and caring for a large house and yard might have contributed to this couple's multiple-year lack of success at conceiving naturally. Greg, a meticulous engineer, used his "only one right answer" skills to map the precise timing of Madison's ovulations. By about the seventh month, however, conceiving a baby took on all too technical aspects. "Living under a microscope is an understatement," he said. "I'm just donor number 082056. Real romantic!"

After nine months of unsuccessful attempts at artificial insemination and countless stressful interactions, the couple came to me to discuss adoption. At the time, I was delivering babies in addition to managing a family practice, and I occasionally had the opportunity to coordinate an adoption. I also gave them the option of trying a course of antibiotics to cure a possible low-grade infection that I have used when all else fails in couples attempting pregnancy. At Greg's request, Madison also cut way back on her work hours. She began working part-time and curtailed her extraneous activities. She had to admit that her stress level declined immensely. The couple each took the antibiotics, and within two months they became pregnant on their own. Ultimately, Madison delivered a healthy baby boy. This was the twelfth couple that had had success with the antibiotic treatment after unsuccessful artificial insemination attempts.

"It was the stress all along," said Greg, bouncing his new baby son on his leg. "We should have recognized the effect of stress and avoided all the cost and hassle of the artificial insemination attempts." And this couple enjoyed a second happy ending: They welcomed a healthy baby girl two years later!

In addition to interfering with conception, a variety of animal and human studies have linked extreme stress and emotional upset to miscarriage. They have shown that increases in adrenaline and noradrenaline can cause decreased blood flow to the uterus, interfering with normal fetal blood supply. Drops in fetal blood pressure and heart rate have been documented in animal studies when mothers are exposed to environmental stressors such as loud noises. Stress also leads to a drop in LH (luteinizing hormone). LH is needed to stimulate the release of progesterone. If sufficient progesterone is not released, the fertilized ovum may not be sustained for the full term. Stress can also lead to poor coping behaviors—such as the increased use of caffeine, alcohol, and tobacco—all detriments to the normal growth and development of a fetus.

Women who have had multiple miscarriages live with almost constant fear, apprehension, and sorrow. They may actually fear becoming pregnant, and this fear increases when they do conceive. Waiting for bleeding or spotting or cramping becomes an overwhelming stressor and causes moment-to-moment anxiety. They monitor every symptom and may miss out on the potential joys of a normal pregnancy.

Biology may drive behavior, but it is far from the only source of stress in your life. In the next chapter we will discuss how these internal stressors combine with external sources of stress to contribute to female stress syndrome.

CHAPTER THREE

Internal and External Stressors: The Vicious Cycle of Chronic Stress

In the previous chapter I explained how the hormones in your body respond to the various stressors in your life, resulting in a cascade of physical, emotional, and behavioral responses beyond your control. But what are the sources of stress in our lives? You might be surprised to learn just how many different kinds of stressors can wreak havoc on your hormone levels.

Some life events may have a stronger stress impact than others. The researchers Thomas Holmes and Richard Rahe, both Ph.D.s, detailed how life stresses can be ranked on a scale from highest to lowest. Their often-cited Social Readjustment Rating Scale, developed in 1968, has been used for years as a screening tool to identify the risk for stress-related illness. Typically, death of a spouse ranks as the worst possible kind of stress and gets a score of 100. Divorce, marital separation, imprisonment, death of a family member, personal injury, and illness all rank in the high-stress category. Marriage, losing a job, marital reconciliation, retirement, change in family member's health, and pregnancy follow as next highest. Sexual difficulties, babies, deaths of friends, changing jobs, owing debts over $10,000, and home foreclosures are lower on the list but still are very stressful events. Children leaving home, starting or stopping work, changes in living conditions, changes in work hours, and changes in religious, recreational, or social activities all contribute to ongoing stress levels. Events that are typically perceived as stressful—such as vacations, Christmas, and minor legal infractions—actually rank lowest on the list.

The factors mentioned are all external stressors. Chronic stress is actually a cycle that feeds on both internal and external factors. These factors can be grouped into seven general categories:

1. Nutritional Stress

Poor nutritional choices can become a major metabolic stress. Nutritional deficiencies, too much protein or fat in your diet, or food allergies can affect your body's stress level and disturb your levels of coping hormones.

One of the resources I recommend to my patients is the book *Toxic Food Syndrome* by Jeffrey Zavik. It discusses the growing body of evidence that certain foods can be toxic, causing undue stress to the body. As the president and CEO of Immuno Laboratories, Zavik has been in the food allergy field since 1978. Evidence from the company's long history of food allergy testing shows that approximately 95% of the U.S. population are allergic to certain foods they eat. Many of the chronic conditions that cause people to seek health care can be attributed to toxic food reactions that cause persistent stress in the body. Symptoms of toxic food allergies vary from person to person and cross the full spectrum of patient complaints.

Food allergy testing can uncover antibodies that we produce in response to certain foods. These antibodies function as a defense mechanism, causing an alarm reaction when certain foods are eaten. The antibodies, called IgG (immunoglobin G) antibodies, surround the gastrointestinal tract and lie in wait for their target food to be eaten. When that happens, the reaction is delayed by several hours to up to three days before symptoms occur. This makes the cause and effect association very elusive to both patients and doctors. For instance, suppose you have undiagnosed IgG antibodies to eggs. You decide to eat an egg. Although you do not experience immediate symptoms, the anti-egg antibody seeks out the egg that you have eaten and causes a cascade of reactions as your body tries to defend itself against this foreign "intruder." Oblivious to the war you have just caused in your intestines, you eat eggs again the next day. The cycle continues, all the while causing many unexplained bodily symptoms.

Sidney Baker, M.D., and his associates at the University of Miami concluded from their study of IgG-reactive foods that eliminating them from the diet reduced the associated symptoms in patients. As a clinician, I have used Immuno Laboratories for food allergy testing, and many of my patients have benefited from knowing which foods their bodies consider to be poison. This was the case with Denise, an attractive teenager with a history of recurrent and severe stomachaches. Her performance in school had been dropping as she missed an increasing number of days due to illness. Her abdominal pain was intermittent, and after multiple doctors and hundreds of dollars of testing and medication trials yielded no definitive diagnosis, Denise and her parents were fed up. "There must be a solution to this problem," her mother said. "But it seems that we have tried nearly everything." Denise added, "I can't tell what causes me to get sick, but it makes me not want to eat at all. I feel better that way." Denise was not talking about an eating disorder, such as an anorexia. She was talking about food allergies. Denise didn't fully understand that what she had eaten two to three days earlier could be causing her current symptoms.

Denise ended up testing positive for over a dozen specific food allergies. Some of the foods, like green beans and kidney beans, were surprises. She also found out that she had antibodies to bananas, which she ate nearly every other day because she thought they would be a healthful food for her! After Denise removed the offending foods from her diet, she felt much better. Her stomach problems became a thing of the past, and her grades rapidly returned to normal. Denise's attitude improved, and her perception of the stress in her life diminished greatly once she was not feeling sick all the time.

Who would have thought that even eating could cause stress? I will help you learn how to avoid problems such as these in step 6 of The Stress Cure.

2. Traumatic Stress

Physical injury such as infection, mechanical injury, burns, or surgery can spark a hormonal fight-or-flight response that can continue even after your physical wounds have healed. The stress from traumatic events can take its toll for weeks, months, and in some cases years after the episode occurs. Many of my patients have told me about traumatic experiences in their lives, stating that they "haven't been the same since."

When trauma occurs, the body goes into instant protection mode. The chemical messages released are intended to amass the biological resources to repair the damage and protect against new offenses. Our body responds to trauma by releasing several stress hormones (for example, norepinephrine, epinephrine). When a person is subjected to repeated or severe trauma, the physiological stress response becomes extreme, and intrusive symptoms of post-traumatic stress disorder (PTSD) can develop. Some studies show that when people who have experienced prolonged or repeated trauma are exposed to any stimulus reminiscent of the trauma, the brain releases opiates (for example, endorphins, enkephalins) that can produce emotional nonresponsiveness, or numbing, and amnesia as a protective mechanism. Serotonin and DHEA depletion may result from repeated exposure to severe stress and trauma, which may be a factor in the development of irritability and violent or angry outbursts in people with PTSD.

Study results published in the January 2002 issue of *Annals of Surgery* suggest that certain female sex hormones play a critical role in maintaining immune responses after trauma. This research showed that female sex hormones decrease the release of TNF-alpha (tumor necrosis factor-alpha) and prevent the increased chance of dying from an overwhelming bacterial infection called sepsis. Thus, maintaining adequate female sex hormones may be useful in preventing a poor immune response after trauma occurs.

Donald Stein, Ph.D., a neuroscientist at Emory University, reports that levels of circulating estrogens and progesterones affect the outcome of brain repair after injury. Women naturally have higher levels of both of these hormones. Studies revealed that when estrogen levels were high, there were many symptoms following brain injury, but when progesterone was high, the symptoms of the same type of injury were not present. Studies of cerebral edema (brain swelling) after trauma reveal a similar protective effect from progesterone in that less swelling was associated with higher progesterone levels and low levels of the hormone caused increased brain swelling. Stein's studies suggest that progesterone plays an active, reparative role in the brain, and he believes it may be possible to use progesterone to protect the brain following such injury. Stein and other researchers suspect that progesterone protects nerves and is a powerful immune system modulator. A growing collection of human research studies support this protective-progesterone theory.

Epidemiologists have found that stroke victims who have yet to go through menopause have better recoveries than postmenopausal women and men (men make much less progesterone than women). Once a woman hits menopause these protective effects disappear. A related series of studies at Memorial Sloan-Kettering Cancer Center in Manhattan showed that breast cancer patients did better—both with regard to recurrence of cancer in the remaining breast and to the risk of dying—if they had undergone surgery during the time in their menstrual cycle when progesterone was high. The higher the progesterone, the better the recovery process. Some doctors are now even experimenting with progesterone treatments for women who have epileptic seizures during a specific phase in their menstrual cycle when estrogen is high. Many of my patients who experience migraine headaches report that their symptoms are more severe or occur only during specific periods of their menstrual cycle. The balance between estrogen and progesterone as well as the influences of cortisol and DHEA clearly play an important role in the immune system.

3. Physical Stress

It should not be surprising that childbirth and hard labor cause physical stress. Inactivity is another physical stressor, but so is excessive exercise, which can weaken your immune system and reduce your resistance to disease.

The good habit of exercise can be carried too far and lead to negative effects, as evidenced by my patient Annette. "Looking back, I realize that the martial arts classes I took last year were probably the cause of my persistent joint pain," she told me. "I always pretended I was really hitting something when I worked out, punching and kicking the air, and I really gave it my all. But you know what they say—No pain no gain!" This was not out of character for Annette, who usually gave her all to everything and everyone. As a result, though, she frequently hyperextended her joints during a vigorous workout. "My joints never hurt while I was doing the activity," she said. "In fact, they felt pretty good." However, the overuse that Annette was inflicting on herself was taking its toll. It took several months of no exercise at all before her joints no longer hurt on a daily basis. Having learned her lesson, Annette then went back to exercising but this time in moderation.

Annette's story is a very common one. With good intentions and high motivation, some women are overexercising, causing stress and strain to their bodies. Other women with too little physical activity in their lives become physically stressed when their bodies need to become active after prolonged periods of inactivity. This is commonly called the weekend warrior syndrome. It can occur in the fall when a brisk wind fills the yard full of leaves. Motivated to clean it all up, the raking marathon begins—and two days later the aches and pains are nearly debilitating. Spring cleaning, painting, or washing the car, walls, or windows may cause repetitive strain syndromes that complicate women's lives. Pain is a message that should be heeded, with appropriate steps taken to diminish it.

4. Chemical Stress

Toxic chemicals, environmental pollution, and certain pharmaceuticals place added stress on your body. Many people are far too complacent about their exposure to these external biological stressors. Today more than

70,000 synthetic chemicals are in commercial use, government research says, with an estimated 1,000 new chemicals being introduced each year. Only a handful of these chemicals have ever been adequately tested to determine their effect on humans and other forms of life (full basic data exists for only about 7% of these chemicals). These toxins and man-made chemicals are in our environment, and we are inadvertently ingesting them daily. Even common substances like caffeine exacerbate the toxic effects associated with stress. Copper pipes, common in home plumbing, can be the source of chemical stress leading to certain associated illnesses.

Many of us may have heard about dioxin. Dioxins are actually a family of 219 different chemicals. Dioxin exposure is a key factor in cancers and reproductive health problems, especially endometriosis and fertility issues in women. Increasingly, women today face a particularly high incidence of reproductive health problems relating to possible environmental chemicals; men's reproductive health is negatively affected as well. Birth defects in newborns may be linked to the mother's environmental exposure to various chemicals during pregnancy.

Here are some facts about the wide-reaching effects of environmental toxins:

- Women whose work exposes them to solvents experience a higher than normal rate of spontaneous abortion (miscarriage).
- Maternal exposure to toluene (used in glues, coatings, inks, and paint) has been shown to cause birth defects.
- Exposure to certain chemicals affecting the endocrine system may have been responsible for a fourfold increase in tubal pregnancies between 1970 and 1987.
- Studies of the umbilical cord blood of newborns have revealed the presence of approximately 100 synthetic chemicals.
- Heart palpitations, insomnia, night sweats, and hormonal imbalances are common signs of chemical poisoning.
- Excessive and recurrent fatigue and other unexplained flu-like symptoms can be triggered by toxic chemicals.
- People prone to headaches often find that a toxic chemical exposure is responsible.
- Unusual skin rashes, swollen glands, digestive problems, nausea, and diarrhea may all be related to toxic poisoning.
- The incidence of symptoms of muscle and joint pain, such as chronic fatigue syndrome and fibromyalgia, is increasing.

- Irritability, aggression, learning disabilities, and behavior disorders may be related to chemical exposure during pregnancy, as well as to persistent exposures after birth.
- Impaired memory, poor concentration, and auditory and visual perception difficulties may be linked to excessive exposure or chronic low-level exposure to toxic chemicals.
- Onset of allergies, asthma, and food, chemical, and noise sensitivity can be traced to acute or chronic exposure to poisons.

Toxic chemicals are introduced into your everyday life in a variety of ways, depending largely on where you live and what activities you do. They are in the air you breathe, the food you eat, and the water you drink. They can readily be found in buildings, in pesticides, and in plenty of consumer products in the home. They are the byproducts of industrial manufacturing, such as the incineration of municipal, medical, and industrial waste; chlorine bleaching processes for paper; pesticide production; and the manufacture of other household and industrial chemicals.

Plastics, some of the main contributors to environmental toxins, contain xenoestrogens, which can have devastating effects on your body's estrogen receptors. Plastic containers, plastic food wrap, plastic soda bottles, and other plastics such as Styrofoam and vinyl products, can release toxins into your food merely by touching it. Heating causes some plastics to break down, releasing toxic substances; hence, microwaving food in containers not meant specifically for high heat, like many disposable food containers, can cause a chemical breakdown and release toxic chemicals into your food.

Several factors determine your risk for illnesses related to toxic exposure. One of the major risk factors is a genetic predisposition to be unable to detoxify certain chemicals and substances that enter your body. Some of us can take higher levels of exposures to various chemicals while others of us cannot. Other factors that influence your response to either acute toxic exposure or sustained chronic toxic exposure include your age, gender, where you live, where you work, activities you do, and your general state of health.

With the advent of affordable genetic testing, you can now find out if you have a genetic predisposition that increases your risk of potential illness from toxic exposures. The ability to detoxify substances is a key component of living a healthy life. Using current testing methods, you can determine if your genes are not coded correctly to produce the detoxifying substances required to get rid of the waste by-products of metabolism and toxic chemicals that have entered your body. Several of my patients have now benefited from tests performed by Great Smokies Diagnostic Laboratory. Several genomic profiles are available, specifically the detoxigenomics profile that uncovers defects in the genetic information telling the body how to detoxify certain substances. After discovering this information, we can work around the genetic error and replace or augment—via nutritional supplementation—that which the body is not making correctly. The ability to uncover an individual's specific genetic mistakes and then provide a natural alternative treatment to essentially correct the deficiency is unprecedented in the history of medicine. The internal stress of not being able to effectively metabolize the toxic chemicals thrust upon us can be greatly diminished when we restore the body's natural defense mechanisms to normal.

Of course, the best way to protect your health is to avoid as many toxins as possible. Here are some ways to reduce your risk of exposure to toxic chemicals:

- Get to know what is in the products you buy for yourself and family.
- Buy organic fruits and vegetables, meats, and dairy products as much as possible.
- Limit your use of products (toilet paper, tampons, and other paper products) that have been subjected to a chlorine process for whitening.
- Limit your exposure to plastic products.
- Use organic pesticides and encourage your neighbors to do the same.

5. Emotional Stress

Anger, depression, fear, frustration, sadness, and bereavement are all forms of emotional stress. Women commonly seek medical treatment for these feelings, but stress is rarely identified as the cause. Instead, many doctors prescribe a myriad of antidepressants and antianxiety agents, counsel their patients to "snap out of it," or comfort the bereaved and urge them to "just give it time."

Chronic strain and lower social power also make women more likely to experience depression. Researchers at the University of Michigan found that the daily strain of work (both in and out of the home) coupled with the feeling of being unappreciated by their partners causes women to feel a great sense of despair that feeds the stress cycle. Feelings of a low sense of control over important areas of their lives fuel feelings of worthlessness. These self-deprecating thoughts continually going around and around in women's minds reinforce depressive feelings and feed the stress response. The result is depression and feelings of hopelessness and helplessness.

The researchers examined 1,100 men and women over a two-year period and found that the women were about twice as likely to be diagnosed with clinical depression as men. They found that "women carried a greater load of the housework and child care and more of the strain of parenting than did men." A common complaint I hear from my female patients was also confirmed in this study as the authors found that women felt less appreciated by their partners than men did. The researchers described a "triad of vulnerabilities" that link women to depression:

- Chronic strain, leading to
- Feelings of helplessness, leading to
- Dwelling on emotions and not taking steps to improve their environments.

The result is a depression that is nearly impossible for a woman to battle on her own. As some women mull over the negative effects of their life situation, they can be drained of the energy needed to make things better. The study reported, "Rumination may maintain chronic strain because it drains people of the motivation, persistence, and problem-solving skills to change their situations." It is no wonder so many women are caught in a web of negativity that causes years of depression and despair.

"We shouldn't just put it on the individual woman to buck up and do something," said Susan Nolen Hoeksema, Ph.D., a psychologist who conducted the study. The solution to the problem is a planned approach; "Helping women achieve a greater sense of control over their circumstances and engage in problem solving rather than ruminating should be useful. Changing the social circumstances that many women face so that they do not have so much to ruminate about is equally important." It is just as important for women's partners as well as business leaders to learn and understand what causes and perpetuates stress in women. Sometimes a very minor adjustment in the environment can make a significant difference in a woman's stress level. Understanding that an improved sense of control over certain areas in a woman's life can dramatically reduce her overall stress levels gives both partners and business associates an opportunity to create better living and working environments.

6. Psychospiritual Stress

This category contains many of what we commonly recognize as stressors: relationships, financial and career pressures, and issues pertaining to life goals. Conflicts regarding spiritual alignment also fall into this category. There are thousands of self-help books available on various aspects of psychospiritual health. In the recommended reading section you'll find several of my personal recommendations for further reading in this fascinating area.

Relationships with others can be one of the most fulfilling and rewarding areas of life. They also can cause a great amount of stress.

My good friend and associate Kevin Connolly, Ph.D., is a clinical psychologist and mental health educator who teaches his patients that having certain expectations that usually go unmet is a setup for increased levels of stress, frustration, and depression. Exploring the issue of expectations and restructuring or loosening your expectations of both yourself and others can help shield you from recurrent feelings of failure and disappointment.

Many of my patients tell me they wake up in the morning, choose to have a good attitude, and begin their day with hope and aspirations. These good feelings rapidly vanish when they turn on the TV and watch the news, listen to the radio, or read the newspaper. "Misery loves company" is a common expression and one that I see played out daily in my patients' lives. Think about all the negative conversations you hear during the course of a typical day. That's why I believe it helps to have nurturing friends and associates who are able to maintain a positive outlook even when times seem tough.

Finances are an extremely high-stress issue for many people, and this trend does not appear to be decreasing. Personal bankruptcies are at an all-time high, and people are in more debt than they have ever been. This ongoing pressure of living on the financial edge is challenging our best intentions to become less stressed. Like quicksand, financial pressures can make you feel as if you are sinking further and further down a deep hole. Avoid the coping mechanism many people use when confronted with financial concerns: "retail therapy." Just as overweight people tend to eat more as a coping mechanism when they are stressed about their excess pounds, so many people attempt to cope with their financial pressures by spending money that they do not have.

7. Mental Stress

Common mental stressors include high responsibility, long hours, anxiety, perfectionism, compulsions, and obsessions. In short, I am referring to a life-sapping lifestyle—the type of lifestyle in which a woman allows daily stresses to mount, leaving her depleted of the vital hormones that help her cope and are essential for feeling "normal." Women adversely affected by their lifestyle are living 24/7 lives, working or worrying 24 hours per day, seven days a week. They multitask: fixing breakfast while preparing their children's lunch, driving to work while talking on a cell phone to a school-teacher, glued to a computer screen at work while also helping the person in the next cubicle do his or her job, trying to care for their husband's emotional needs while ignoring their own. They can never focus on one thing because two or more things need to be done at the same time. Such women report feeling "drained," an appropriate word since stress is literally draining them of estrogen, progesterone, testosterone, and DHEA, the hormones that allow them to cope. In addition, the neurotransmitter serotonin can become depleted by a frenetic lifestyle, causing increased feelings of anxiety.

America's working women have been hit particularly hard by the stress epidemic. A 2000 survey sponsored by the AFL-CIO reported that these women feel stressed out and overwhelmed: 60% worked 40 or more hours a week. Of those with children under 18, half worked different shifts from their spouses or partners. A Duke University study concurred, finding that working women with children have higher levels of stress hormones than women without children, and a University of Iowa study reported that workaholics have more conflicts between work and family and less satisfaction and purpose in life.

This constant battle between responsibilities in and out of the home is a major stressor for women of the twenty-first century. Often, impelled by the need for increased household income, women are pushed to work outside the home. With high taxes and debt load increasing the financial burden on families today, however, the added income is relative and in actuality can be much less than initially perceived. This scenario causes a common feeling of defeat in many women and their partners. What was originally thought of as a financial benefit that should improve self-esteem via increased productivity leads to feelings of frustration and disappointment. When these feelings of sadness, frustration, and being overwhelmed well up, some women respond by working harder, only adding to their already overworked, undernurtured lifestyle. Jody, one of my patients, accurately describes this pattern: "When I come home at night, I am totally exhausted. I walk in the door and within seconds I am bombarded with questions from my children. I haven't even put the groceries down and I am answering questions about the next weekend. I instantly feel panic race through my body, and a wave of emotion washes over me as I take a deep breath and focus on putting the groceries away. 'I can't think about the weekend right now.' 'We'll do your homework after dinner.' 'Please pick up your clothes and make your bed,' I request as I am running up the stairs to put away the new toothpaste and shampoo. I just keep myself busy when I get those feelings; otherwise I collapse and start crying—and can't stop. Sometimes I just want to run away from all the responsibilities. I feel like no one even knows or appreciates all that I do for them. When is it *my* turn?" Jody works about 50 hours a week and always has an immaculate home. She is first to work and last to leave. She "does it all"—at tremendous personal cost.

The Result

The seven types of stresses can come at us from all sides of life, having a cumulative effect and interfering with the natural balance of hormones and neurotransmitters. But that doesn't mean that everyone is affected by all seven types of stress at one time. Each of us is affected by a unique combination of internal and external stressors. What's more, a person's stress profile changes over time, depending on hormone levels, lifestyle, nutrition, and all the other factors mentioned in this chapter.

So how do you identify your own personal stressors? The next chapter contains a self-assessment tool to help you learn more about where your own stress comes from. Once you better understand the sources of your stress, you will be able to target The Stress Cure to address your own, unique needs.

CHAPTER FOUR

Dr. Vern's Stress Cure Inventory: A Self-Assessment

After reading the first three chapters of this book, you probably know more about stress than you ever have. You may have recognized yourself in some of the cases. Now it's time to personalize the De-STRESS program to fit *your* unique situation.

The first step is to learn exactly where your stress is coming from. This chapter contains a questionnaire called Dr. Vern's Stress Cure Inventory. It contains 60 questions on such topics as nutritional supplements; stress reduction techniques, coping abilities, locus of control, and fear and anxiety; relationships and sexuality; work (both in the home and outside the home); exercise, fatigue, and somatic complaints; eating patterns; and sleep patterns.

This self-graded questionnaire will give you a clearer understanding of the level of stress you are experiencing and how that stress is manifesting itself in your daily life. Record your responses on a separate sheet of paper. After a few months on The Stress Cure, take the assessment again and compare your scores. See how much your responses have changed.

This process can be very helpful in judging improvements in your stress levels and gauging your ongoing progress. As you regain control of your life, it is very important to remain in the driver's seat. Think of this self-assessment as one of the instruments on your control panel.

Seven Steps to Success

Dr. Vern's Stress Cure Inventory was developed as a tool to help you identify those areas in your life that may be functioning quite well and others that may need significant attention. The questions cover a spectrum of health-related issues that are intimately involved in building up or tearing down your stress defenses. Don't be alarmed if you feel apprehensive as you complete the survey. You probably wouldn't be reading this book if everything in your life was purring along perfectly! Remember, this process is for you. Just be honest with yourself. You are not out to impress anyone. You are just taking your current "stress temperature" before you take steps to move on to a greater sense of well-being. As mentioned, you can take the questionnaire over and over again to watch yourself improve as you proceed through The Stress Cure.

This questionnaire will set the foundation and prepare you for steps 2–7 of The Stress Cure. These six steps, in addition to refueling your DHEA levels, will ignite your ability to reduce and control the major sources of stress in your life:

- Supplemental Nutrition (questions 1–10)
- Taming the Tiger (questions 11–20)
- Rekindling Relationships (questions 21–30)
- Effective Exercising (questions 31–40)
- Sensible Eating (questions 41–50)
- Sound Sleep (questions 51–60)

SUPPLEMENTAL NUTRITION

Contrary to nearly everything I was taught in traditional medical school, the need to supplement your daily nutrition in order to attain optimal health is becoming more obvious every day, as research confirms what many nutritional health practitioners have been saying for years. It is exciting and rewarding to experience the growth and appreciation of functional medicine and nutritional biochemistry that is occurring in the field of medicine today. Nutritional recommendations that were once considered quackery are now considered malpractice if they are not prescribed as a matter of course. Folic acid, given in pregnancy to avoid major birth defects, is a perfect example.

The following 10 questions will give you an idea of the understanding you have and priority you place on nutrition and nutrional supplments. A point value appears beside each possible response.

1. **On average, how many glasses of water do you consume per day?**
    1) I seldom consume water.
    2) I drink 1–2 glasses, 8 oz each, per day.
    3) I drink 3–4 glasses, 8 oz each, per day.
    4) I drink 5–6 glasses, 8 oz each, per day.
    5) I drink 7–8 glasses, 8 oz each, per day.

2. **How many servings of alcoholic beverages do you consume daily?**
    1) I drink more than 3 glasses of wine or 3 cans/bottles of beer or 3 alcoholic drinks per day.
    2) I drink 2–3 glasses of wine or 2–3 cans of beer or 2–3 alcoholic drinks per day.
    3) I drink 1 glass of wine or 1 can/bottle of beer or 1 alcoholic drink per day.
    4) I rarely consume alcohol other than on special/infrequent occasions.
    5) I never consume alcohol.

3. **How many servings of caffeinated beverages (sodas, coffee, or tea) do you consume daily?**
    1) I drink more than 5 caffeinated drinks per day.
    2) I drink 4–5 caffeinated drinks per day.
    3) I drink 2–3 caffeinated drinks per day.
    4) I drink 0–1 caffeinated drinks per day.
    5) I never consume caffeine.

4. **What kind of multivitamins do you take each day?**
    1) I do not take a multivitamin supplement.
    2) I usually take an inexpensive or "discount" multivitamin daily.

3) I usually take a regular or "retail" multivitamin daily.

4) I usually take 1–3 high-quality multivitamins daily.

5) I usually take 4 or more high-quality multivitamins daily.

5. **How many antioxidant supplements do you take daily?**

1) I do not know what an antioxidant is and do not take any.

2) I know what an antioxidant is but do not take any.

3) I take a single antioxidant, such as vitamin C or E, occasionally.

4) I take a single antioxidant, such as vitamin C or E, daily.

5) I take a multiple-combination antioxidant formulation daily.

6. **What is your daily intake of the minerals chromium, magnesium, and selenium?**

1) I haven't heard of chromium, magnesium, or selenium.

2) I know the value of these minerals but do not take them as a supplement.

3) I take 1 of the minerals listed above as a daily supplement.

4) I take 2 of the minerals listed above as a daily supplement.

5) I take all 3 of the minerals listed above as a daily supplement.

7) **How much vitamin C do you use as a daily nutritional supplement?**

1) Vitamin C is overrated, and I don't take any extra as a supplement.

2) I try to drink a glass of juice or beverage with vitamin C daily.

3) I take a small amount of vitamin C (less than 500 mg) daily.

4) I take a moderate amount of vitamin C (500 mg–1,000 mg) daily.

5) I take a large amount of vitamin C (more than 1,000 mg) daily.

8. How much folic acid/folate, do you use as a daily nutritional supplement?
    1) I do not know about folic acid and do not take any extra as a supplement.
    2) I have heard about the benefits of folic acid but do not take any extra.
    3) I take a small amount of folic acid/folate (100 mcg) daily.
    4) I take a moderate amount of folic acid/folate (400 mcg) daily.
    5) I take a large amount of folic acid/folate (800 mcg) daily.

9. What is your daily intake of vitamin B_5 (pantothenic acid)?
    1) I do not take any extra vitamin B_5/pantothenic acid.
    2) I take vitamin B_5/pantothenic acid on an occasional basis once per week.
    3) I take vitamin B_5/pantothenic acid on an occasional basis 3 times per week.
    4) I take vitamin B_5/pantothenic acid on a daily basis.
    5) I take vitamin B complex containing vitamin B_5 on a daily basis.

10. What is your daily intake of coenzyme Q10?
    1) I have never heard of coenzyme Q10 or what it does.
    2) I do not take any extra coenzyme Q10 on a daily basis.
    3) I take coenzyme Q10 on an occasional basis once per week.
    4) I take coenzyme Q10 on an occasional basis 3 times per week.
    5) I take coenzyme Q10 on a daily basis.

Add the point values of your answers from all 10 questions in this section. The maximum points in this section are 50.

Total Score This Section _____

- If you scored 41–50 points, you are doing an excellent job. You probably put nutritional supplementation high on your priority list.
- If you scored 31–40 points, you are doing well and know that nutri-

tional supplementation is important, but you would probably feel much better by placing more emphasis on making better choices.

- If you scored 21–30 points, you are probably not placing much emphasis on nutritional supplementation and could be putting your health at risk and increasing the stress on your body.
- If you scored 10–20 points, you are putting little effort toward nutritional supplementation and you may be severely challenging your body's ability to respond to stress adequately. Consider this a wake-up call.

TAMING THE TIGER

Stress is a tiger that is hard to tame for many people. The following 10 questions will help you identify how successful you are at using known stress reduction techniques. They will help you understand the priority you place on decreasing the level of stress in your life.

11. How often do you set limits on the commitments you make?
  1) I never set limits; I always take on more than I can possibly do.
  2) I try to set limits but I am not very effective. I always have more than I can possibly do.
  3) I will set limits and usually get most things accomplished, but when given a choice I will do for others at my own expense.
  4) I will set limits and usually get everything accomplished, but I would like more time for my personal responsibilities.
  5) I have a healthy balance between commitments to others and commitments to myself.

12. How often do you feel overwhelmed?
  1) Constantly—24 hours a day, 7 days a week.
  2) I nearly always feel overwhelmed—about 80% of the time.
  3) I usually feel overwhelmed—about 50% of the time.
  4) I occasionally feel overwhelmed—about 20% of the time.
  5) I rarely feel overwhelmed—about 5% of the time.

13. **How often do you feel as though feel things are out of control?**
    1) Several times a day.
    2) At least once a day.
    3) At least once a week.
    4) At least once a month.
    5) I never feel out of control.

14. **How much personal control do you feel you have over your life?**
    1) I never feel I have control over what happens to me.
    2) I rarely feel I have control over what happens to me.
    3) I sometimes feel I have control over what happens to me.
    4) I usually feel I have control over what happens to me.
    5) I always feel I have control over what happens to me.

15. **How much responsibility do you have for your home environment?**
    1) 100%
    2) 75%
    3) 50%
    4) 25%
    5) 10%

16. **How often do you actively try to reduce the stress in your life?**
    1) I never try to reduce stress; I can't do anything about it.
    2) I try to reduce stress but in unhealthy ways (for example, alcohol).
    3) I am occasionally active at reducing stress through healthy solutions.
    4) I am usually active at reducing stress through healthy solutions.
    5) I am very active at reducing stress through healthy solutions.

17. **How often do you take a relaxing bath?**
    1) Almost never.
    2) Occasionally—once every 3 months.
    3) Monthly.

    4) Weekly.

    5) Daily.

18. **How often do you read purely for enjoyment?**
    1) Almost never.
    2) Occasionally—once a month.
    3) Once per week.
    4) 15–30 minutes per day.
    5) 30–60 minutes or more per day.

19. **How often do you worry about your financial status?**
    1) I worry about finances all the time; I'm always behind with bills.
    2) I worry all the time; some bills are overdue.
    3) I usually worry about finances, but all bills are paid.
    4) I occasionally worry about finances, but all bills are paid.
    5) I never worry; I feel confident about my financial status.

20. **How easily are you able to ask others for help?**
    1) I would never burden others with my problems or needs.
    2) I rarely ask others for help, and when I do I feel guilty.
    3) I occasionally ask others for help, but I feel I should have been able to handle things myself.
    4) I will ask others for help as a last resort, understanding that I can't do everything.
    5) I have no problem asking others for help when it is appropriate.

Add the point values of your answers from all 10 questions in this section. The maximum points in this section are 50.

Total Score This Section _____

- If you scored 41–50 points, you are doing an excellent job. You are probably putting stress reduction techniques high on your priority list.

- If you scored 31–40 points, you are doing well and know that reducing stress is important. You could probably feel much better by placing more emphasis on making better choices.
- If you scored 21–30 points, you are probably not placing much emphasis on taming your stress tiger and could be significantly putting your health at risk.
- If you scored 10–20 points, you are putting little effort toward stress reduction, and you may be severely challenging your body's ability to respond to stress adequately. Consider this a wake-up call.

REKINDLING RELATIONSHIPS

The need to cultivate and nurture close relationships is an essential human instinct. The energy among friends and loved ones can warm any stressful situation. At times of stress we tend to invest less time and energy in these close relationships because we are constantly pressed for time and mental energy. We often neglect those who are the closest to us because other obligations seem to take priority.

The following 10 questions will help you identify how successful you are at doing the things that keep relationships growing, and how much priority you give them.

21. **How social are you with other people?**
1) I have no interest in being social.
2) I have lost much interest in all but a few people.
3) I try not to be around many people, as they usually annoy me.
4) I'm interested in being around people but am sometimes annoyed by them.
5) I'm very interested in people and enjoy being around them.

22. **How do you feel about the relationship with your spouse or significant other?**
1) I have no relationship right now.
2) Our relationship is getting worse.
3) Our relationship is flat, on average—with some ups, some downs.

4) Our relationship is pretty good.

5) Our relationship is excellent.

23. **How easy is it to talk with your spouse or significant other?**

    1) I have no spouse or significant other.

    2) It is difficult—doesn't listen, usually defensive.

    3) It is not easy—rarely listens, usually defensive.

    4) It is fairly easy—usually listens, sometimes defensive.

    5) It is very easy—always listens without being defensive.

24. **How much high-quality time do you spend with your spouse or significant other?**

    1) I have no spouse or significant other.

    2) We spend quality time about one hour a month.

    3) We spend quality time about one hour per week.

    4) We spend quality time several hours per week.

    5) We usually spend several hours of quality time every day.

25. **How often do you have verbal arguments with your spouse or significant other?**

    1) Frequently, almost daily.

    2) At least once a week.

    3) At least once a month.

    4) About once every three months.

    5) I can't remember the last time we verbally argued.

26. **How is your relationship with others in your family?**

    1) Very strained—they aggravate me all the time.

    2) Tolerable if I don't have to see them too much.

    3) OK—nothing really positive or negative.

    4) My family makes me feel good most of the time.

    5) My family is nurturing, and spending time with them makes me feel great.

27. **How is your sex life (including sexual desire)?**

    1) What sex life? It doesn't exist, and I don't want it to.

    2) I provide "courtesy sex," but otherwise I could take it or leave it.

3) I have a low libido, am rarely aroused, and sometimes enjoy sex.

4) I have a moderate libido, am usually aroused, and usually enjoy sex.

5) I have a great libido, am easily aroused, and frequently enjoy sex.

28. **Do you feel acknowledged or appreciated by your family?**
    1) I never feel acknowledged or appreciated.
    2) I rarely feel acknowledged or appreciated.
    3) I sometimes feel acknowledged or appreciated.
    4) I usually feel acknowledged or appreciated.
    5) I always feel acknowledged or appreciated.

29. **How is your relationship with your work? (Score 3 if you do not work outside the home.)**
    1) Work is very stressful and intolerable most of the time.
    2) Work is very stressful but I can usually tolerate it.
    3) Work is stressful but tolerable most of the time.
    4) Work is stressful but I usually enjoy it.
    5) Work is sometimes stressful but fulfilling, and I enjoy it.

30. **How is your relationship with yourself?**
    1) I am extremely self-critical and always hard on myself.
    2) I am very self-critical and usually hard on myself.
    3) I am self-critical and sometimes hard on myself.
    4) I feel positive about myself and occasionally am hard on myself.
    5) I feel very positive about myself and rarely am hard on myself.

Add the point values of your answers from all 10 questions in this section. The maximum points on this section are 50.

Total Score This Section _____

• If you scored 41–50 points, you are doing an excellent job and probably put the importance of relationships high on your priority list.

- If you scored 31–40 points, you are doing well. You could probably feel much better by making some changes in how you relate to people.
- If you scored 21–30 points, you are probably not placing much emphasis on your relationships and could be significantly putting your health at risk and increasing the stress on your body.
- If you scored 10–20 points, you are putting little effort toward good relationships, and you may be severely challenging your body's ability to respond to stress. Consider this a wake-up call.

EFFECTIVE EXERCISING

Never in human history have we been more sedentary. With the advent of the remote control and the personal computer, as well as many other creature comforts, we sit for long periods of time. The increased inactivity is causing Americans to put on weight at exponential rates. Obesity is at an all-time high and getting higher every year, with the incidence of serious diseases such as diabetes rising right along with it. The most recent studies report that up to 60% of the U.S. population is overweight, and the obesity epidemic is extending into childhood. Currently over 13% of children and 16% of adolescents in the United States are overweight. Large amounts of calorie-dense fast foods combined with a lack of effective exercise can cause tremendous negative stress and deconditioning in the body. Recent research published in the October 2002 issue of the *New England Journal of Medicine* found that as little as three weeks of aggressive exercise begins to lower cardiac risk factors. It's never too late to begin to restore your health and vitality. Are you exercising enough? The following questions will help you find out.

31. **On average, how many days do you walk as exercise for 30 minutes per day?**
    1) I never walk specifically to exercise.
    2) I walk 1–2 days per week.
    3) I walk 3–4 days per week.
    4) I walk 5–6 days per week.
    5) I walk every day for 30 minutes or more.

32. **On average, how much upper-extremity weight training do you do?**
    1) I do no upper-extremity weight training.
    2) I do upper-extremity weight training 1 day per month.
    3) I do upper-extremity weight training 1 day per week.
    4) I do upper-extremity weight training 3 days per week.
    5) I do upper-extremity weight training daily.

33. **On average, how much lower-extremity weight training do you do?**
    1) I do no lower-extremity weight training.
    2) I do lower-extremity weight training 1 day per month.
    3) I do lower-extremity weight training 1 day per week.
    4) I do lower-extremity weight training 3 days per week.
    5) I do lower-extremity weight training daily.

34. **On average, how much aerobic activity do you engage in?**
    1) I do no aerobic activity.
    2) I do aerobic activity 1 day per month.
    3) I do aerobic activity 1 day per week.
    4) I do aerobic activity 3 days per week.
    5) I do aerobic activity daily.

35. **How do you experience the relationship between stress and exercise?**
    1) I feel stressed because I never exercise.
    2) I rarely exercise, and it is stressful to do so.
    3) I exercise monthly, and it would help me if I did more.
    4) I exercise weekly and know it helps reduce my stress.
    5) I exercise daily and know it helps reduce my stress.

36. **How is your energy level?**
    1) What energy? I am exhausted all the time.
    2) I have very low energy; I am frequently exhausted.
    3) I have a poor energy level but am rarely exhausted.
    4) I have a good energy level, but I am occasionally exhausted.
    5) I have a great energy level; I am rarely exhausted.

37. **What is the level of pain in your joints?**
    1) All of my major joints hurt all of the time.
    2) All of my joints hurt most of the time.
    3) I have joint pain that occurs daily.
    4) I have joint pain that occurs weekly.
    5) I rarely have joint pain.

38. **How would you describe your overall activity level?**
    1) I am very sedentary.
    2) I am somewhat inactive.
    3) I am usually active.
    4) I am very active.
    5) I am extremely active.

39. **How often to you practice yoga, tai chi, or a similar activity?**
    1) I never practice such activities.
    2) I practice such activities 1 day per month.
    3) I practice such activities 1 day per week.
    4) I practice such activities 3 days per week.
    5) I practice such activities daily.

40. **How do you feel about fitting exercise into your life?**
    1) I have no time or interest in exercising.
    2) It may be important, but I can't find the time to
       do it.
    3) Exercise is important. I am not doing enough now; I
       may try to do more.
    4) Exercise is very important. I am not doing enough now;
       I will definitely arrange to do more.
    5) Exercise is critically important. I exercise adequately and
       will continue to do so.

Add the point values of your answers from all 10 questions in this section. The maximum points in this section are 50.

Total Score This Section _____

• If you scored 41–50 points, you are doing an excellent job and probably put exercising high on your priority list.

- If you scored 31–40 points, you are doing well and know that exercise is important, but could probably feel much better by placing more emphasis on making better choices.
- If you scored 21–30 points, you are probably not placing much emphasis on physical fitness and could be significantly putting your health at risk and increasing the stress on your body.
- If you scored 10–20 points, you are putting little effort toward physical exercise or cardiac conditioning, and you may be severely challenging your body's ability to respond to stress adequately. Consider this a wake-up call.

SENSIBLE EATING

"The cornerstone to your health is diet," says Framingham Heart Study director William Castelli, M.D. The Framingham Heart Study was a 24-year observational analysis of nearly 6,000 patients, focusing on lifestyle and health habits. The study's conclusions supported many nutritional experts' recommendations about the food we choose to consume. What we eat provides the nutrients our body uses to fuel each and every one of our cells. Our diets determine how vigorous we feel, how well we respond to daily stressors, and how easily we are able to repair problems in our bodies when they occur. In some of us, our diets can contribute significantly to the added stress our body is under and can worsen, rather than help, our ability to deal with stress.

It is sad to note that less than one-third of all Americans meet the government's Healthy People 2000 goal of eating five or more servings of fruits and vegetables per day. Most people only eat only 1.2 servings of fruit and 3.1 servings of vegetables daily, according to the *American Journal of Public Health*. Are you providing your body with the best and the most appropriate fuel it needs to respond to stress, maintain health, and optimize energy? Answer the following ten questions to find out.

41. **Are you interested in nutrition and its effects on the body?**
    1) I have very little interest in nutrition. I eat anything and everything.
    2) I agree that some foods are bad for me but say, "what the heck."

3) I understand that nutrition has a very important influence on how I feel. I try to eat healthy foods, but I'm usually not successful.

4) I understand that nutrition is vitally important and more often than not eat nutritionally healthy foods.

5) I understand nutrition is critical to my well-being and almost always eat nutritionally healthy foods.

42. Are you currently overweight (using ideal body weight for females as 100 pounds for the first 5 feet of height and adding 5 pounds for every inch above that, for example, 5 feet 5 inches = 125 pounds)?

1) I am more than 30 pounds over my ideal body weight.

2) I am within 30 pounds of my ideal body weight.

3) I am within 15 pounds of my ideal body weight.

4) I am within 5 pounds of my ideal body weight.

5) I am currently at my ideal body weight.

43. On average, how many meals do you consume per day?

1) I have no regular eating pattern; I usually eat fast food.

2) I usually eat 2 meals or less per day; I frequently eat fast food.

3) I usually eat 3 meals per day; I occasionally eat fast food.

4) I eat 3 meals per day. They are usually well-balanced, rarely fast food.

5) I eat 3–6 well-balanced meals per day. I almost never eat fast foods."

44. On average, how much meat (or meat products) do you consume per day?

1) I consume red meats early every day.

2) I consume red meats regularly, at least 1–3 times per week.

3) I consume red meats rarely but eat poultry or fish nearly daily.

4) I do not eat red meat and consume poultry or fish occasionally.

5) I do not consume any meat or meat products.

45. **On average, how many servings of fats, dressings, and spreads do you consume per day?**
    1) I eat high-fat selections frequently, more than 3 times per day.
    2) I eat high-fat selections sparingly, less than 3 times per day.
    3) I eat low-fat and high-fat selections sparingly, about 3 times per day.
    4) I eat low-fat selections frequently, 3 or more times a day.
    5) I eat low-fat selections sparingly, less than 3 times a day.

46. **On average, how many dairy products do you consume per day?**
    1) I eat high-fat dairy products frequently, more than 5 times per day.
    2) I eat high-fat dairy products frequently, 3–5 times per day.
    3) I eat high-fat dairy products sparingly, less than 3 times per day.
    4) I eat low-fat dairy products frequently, 3 or more times per day.
    5) I eat low-fat dairy products sparingly, less than 3 times per day.

47. **On average, how many vegetables do you eat each day?**
    1) I hardly ever eat vegetables.
    2) I eat 1–2 servings of vegetables per day.
    3) I eat 3–4 servings of vegetables per day.
    4) I eat 5 servings of vegetables per day, usually cooked.
    5) I eat 5 servings of vegetables per day, often uncooked.

48. **How many servings of whole grain bread products do you consume daily?**
    1) I rarely consume grain products.
    2) I consume more than 6 servings daily of refined grains such as white rolls, white bread.
    3) I consume 1–6 servings daily of refined grains.
    4) I consume 1–6 servings daily of whole grains.
    5) I consume more than 6 servings daily of whole grains.

49. **How many servings of beans, peas, or legumes do you eat daily?**
    1) What is a legume?
    2) I follow no regular eating pattern of beans, peas, or legumes.
    3) I usually eat beans, peas, or legumes once per a day.
    4) I usually eat beans, peas, or legumes 2 times per day.
    5) I usually eat beans, peas, or legumes 3 or more times per day.

50. **On average, how much refined carbohydrate (sugar, candy, cakes, cookies, etc.) do you consume per day?**
    1) I consume more than 6 servings per day.
    2) I consume 5–6 servings per day.
    3) I consume 3–4 servings per day.
    4) I consume 1–2 servings per day.
    5) I seldom consume refined carbohydrates.

Add the point values of your answers from all 10 questions in this section. The maximum points on this section are 50.

Total Score This Section _____

- If you scored 41–50 points, you are doing an excellent job and probably put sensible eating high on your priority list.
- If you scored 31–40 points, you are doing well and know that eating appropriately is important but could probably feel much better by placing more emphasis on making better choices.
- If you scored 21–30 points, you are probably not placing much emphasis on good eating habits and could be significantly putting your health at risk and increasing the stress on your body.
- If you scored 10–20 points, you are putting little effort toward eating sensibly, and you may be severely challenging your body's ability to respond to stress adequately. Consider this a wake-up call.

SOUND SLEEP

Insomnia, which affects 49% of the American population, is largely due to stress and anxiety. Of adults who experience occasional insomnia, 79% have trouble sleeping an average of 6 nights per month, and 26% have difficulty averaging 16 nights per month. The majority of sufferers never discuss the problem with their physicians; only 6% seek medical attention for sleep difficulties.

Lack of sleep can make our problems and stresses seem much greater than they really are. Inadequate sleep lowers cognitive abilities and neuro-muscular control, causes forgetfulness and difficulty in forming new memories, and also literally puts our lives in danger. A 1998 survey by the National Sleep Foundation found that an astonishing 30% of men and 15% of women reported falling asleep while driving within the prior year. Answer the following questions to see how soundly you are sleeping.

51. **How well do you fall asleep when retiring for the night?**
    1) I lie awake for 2 hours or more.
    2) I lie awake for 1–2 hours.
    3) I lie awake for 30 minutes to an hour.
    4) I usually fall asleep by 30 minutes.
    5) I easily fall asleep within a few minutes.

52. **How well do you sleep throughout the night?**
    1) I experience 5 or more interruptions per night.
    2) I experience 4 interruptions per night.
    3) I experience 3 interruptions per night.
    4) I experience 1–2 interruptions per night.
    5) I do not experience sleep interruptions during the night.

53. **On average, how much sleep do you get a night?**
    1) I sleep less than two hours per night.
    2) I sleep 2–3 hours per night.
    3) I sleep 4–5 hours per night.
    4) I sleep 5–7 hours per night.
    5) I sleep 7–9 hours per night.

54. **How good is your memory?**
    1) I frequently have memory problems, and they are getting worse.
    2) I frequently have memory problems, but they are not changing.
    3) I often have memory problems that are made worse when I don't sleep.
    4) I occasionally have memory problems that are made worse when I don't sleep.
    5) I rarely have memory problems.

55. **How do you feel after a night's rest?**
    1) I am exhausted all of the time whether I sleep or not.
    2) I feel tired when I wake up and remain tired most of the day.
    3) I feel good for a few hours but get tired early in the day and tire easily.
    4) I feel energetic at the beginning of the day but get tired toward the end of the day.
    5) I feel energetic most of the time.

56. **Do you feel your mood is related to the quality of sleep you get?**
    1) My mood is generally bad, and it is worse when I don't sleep well.
    2) My mood is usually OK, but it turns bad when I don't sleep well.
    3) My mood is generally good but can turn bad when I don't sleep well.
    4) My mood is usually great but gets worse when I don't sleep well.
    5) My mood is great and is not affected when I don't sleep well.

57. **What is your understanding of melatonin?**
    1) I have no idea what melatonin is.
    2) I have heard about melatonin but do not know what it is.
    3) I understand that melatonin is found in every living substance.

4) I understand that melatonin is secreted at different levels throughout the day and may be the trigger that puts us to sleep and wakes us up.

5) I understand that melatonin is made from an essential amino acid called tryptophan, which is converted into 5-hydroxytryptophan, then serotonin, and finally into melatonin.

58. **Which of the following best describes you?**

1) I am depressed and anxious, and I consume alcohol and/or illegal drugs frequently to relax and help me sleep.

2) I am depressed and anxious, and I consume alcohol and/or prescription drugs frequently to relax and help me sleep.

3) I am depressed and anxious, and I consume alcohol and/or prescription drugs occasionally to relax and help me sleep.

4) I am depressed and anxious. I use nothing to help me relax and sleep.

5) I am not depressed or anxious. I sleep well.

59. **How many of the following problems do you experience during your sleep periods: snoring/sleep apnea, restless legs syndrome, frequent awakening, night sweats, jaw clenching/teeth grinding?**

1) I experience 4 or more of the above.

2) I experience 3 of the above.

3) I experience 2 of the above.

4) I experience 1 of the above.

5) I experience none of the above.

60. **What is your understanding of sleep and its protection of the brain? (Choose the highest answer that best describes you.)**

1) I did not know that sleep actually helps protect the brain.

2) I know very little about the protective effects of sleep on the brain.

3) I understand that the benefits of sleep are probably influenced by factors such as growth hormone.

4) I understand that sleep functions like an antioxidant for the brain because free radicals are removed during this time, when growth hormone is maximally secreted.

5) I understand that as we age we get less sleep and therefore we secrete less growth hormone to scavenge free
radicals, causing brain degeneration to accelerate, leading
to a decline in mental functioning.

Add the point values of your answers from all 10 questions in this
section. The maximum points on this section are 50.

Total Score This Section _____

- If you scored 41–50 points, you are doing an excellent job and
  probably put good sleep hygiene high on your priority list.
- If you scored 31–40 points, you are doing well and know that a
  good night's sleep is important but could probably feel much better by placing more emphasis on making better choices.
- If you scored 21–30 points, you are probably not placing much
  emphasis on good sleep habits and could be significantly putting
  your health at risk and increasing the stress on your body.
- If you scored 10–20 points, you are putting little effort toward
  sleeping soundly, and you may be severely challenging your
  body's ability to respond to stress adequately. Consider this a
  wake-up call.

THE STRESS CURE INVENTORY SUMMARY

Now it's time to total your score for all six sections. Remember that each
question has a maximum of five points, each section a maximum of 50
points, and the maximum total of all six sections is 300 points. Total your
scores from all six sections below.

Supplemental Nutrition	(questions 1–10)	_____
Taming the Tiger	(questions 11–20)	_____
Rekindling Relationships	(questions 21–30)	_____
Effective Exercising	(questions 31–40)	_____
Sensible Eating	(questions 41–50)	_____
Sound Sleep	(questions 51–60)	_____

Total Points _____

- If you scored 240–300 points, you are doing an excellent job and probably put nutritional supplements, stress reduction techniques, relationships, exercise, sensible eating, and sleeping soundly high on your priority list.
- If you scored 180–239 points, you are doing well and know that all of these factors are important but could probably feel much better by placing more emphasis on making better choices.
- If you scored 120–179 points, you are probably not placing much emphasis on many of these factors and could be significantly putting your health at risk and increasing the stress on your body.
- If you scored 60–119 points, you are putting little effort toward enhancing your nutrition with supplements, taming the tiger by stress reduction, rekindling relationships with others, exercising adequately, eating sensibly, and sleeping soundly. You may be severely challenging your body's ability to respond to stress adequately. Consider this a wake-up call.

Now That You Know

Now that you have completed The Stress Cure Inventory, you should have an excellent idea of just how high your stress level is and which parts of your life are causing you the biggest problems. You should also be able to identify areas of opportunity where you can modify your lifestyle. You may have learned some ways you are harming your body without even knowing it. Changing these behaviors can make a big difference in how your body responds to the stresses in your life and, ultimately, how well you feel on a daily basis.

Now that you have a good idea of where you are "stressologically," you are ready to move on to Part II of The Stress Cure to learn about the seven steps to De-STRESS.

PART II

The Stress Cure: Seven Steps to "De-STRESS"

CHAPTER FIVE

Step 1: Dehydroepiandrosterone

The first step in The Stress Cure is supplemental DHEA. But before you start taking DHEA supplements, you should know what your untreated DHEA levels are.

DHEA can be measured using either blood or saliva. There are also two forms of DHEA that can be evaluated. Technically, DHEA refers to the free, or "unbound," form of the hormone. DHEA-S, the sulfated, or "storage," form of DHEA, reflects the reservoir of DHEA available to the body to be activated when needed. Free, or unbound, DHEA is short-lived in the blood (around 30 minutes) and is either used, converted to other metabolic compounds, or sulfated and put into the storage form, DHEA-S. Both DHEA and DHEA-S levels can be tested, and each form has its own characteristics.

I usually order a DHEA-S level on my patients via a blood (serum) sample because I like to evaluate their total body storage form of DHEA. DHEA levels tested via saliva are less stable than DHEA-S serum levels. I also prefer to test for DHEA-S because it reflects the total body reserve, or total body status, of DHEA available for activation. I am concerned when the total body stores are low even if the active form is in the normal range.

I rarely see women not taking a DHEA supplement with a DHEA-S level approaching a good or excellent number. Most are either low or in the serious deficiency category. Many patients I have treated who are suffering from female stress syndrome have DHEA values well under 50 ng/dl. Some patients have DHEA-S levels that are *undetectable* by laboratory testing.

DHEA Reference Values

The following tables list normal ranges for DHEA and DHEA-S blood levels for men and women. The most common units of measure are nanograms per deciliter (ng/dl) for unbound DHEA and micrograms per deciliter (mcg/dl μ) for DHEA-S. Table 5.1 reports the blood levels for free, or unbound, DHEA. Table 5.2 reports the blood levels for DHEA-S, the sulfated, storage form of DHEA. (Be aware that different laboratories use different reporting formats, and each lab may have a specific set of reference values that correspond to their particular testing equipment. This means that "normal" values may differ slightly between labs. It is important to evaluate your own reported values against the reference values of the laboratory performing your tests with the help of your personal physician).

It is also important to note that the broad range of values in the "normal" or "reference" range may not be indicative of the *best* level for *your* personal optimum health and well-being. Many health care practitioners will report to you that your "levels are fine—in the normal range." There are several factors that should be considered in determining what DHEA level is the best for you and what level you should try to achieve. This is best decided in cooperation with a health care provider who is aware of the benefits of DHEA and is comfortable using this natural supplement as part of your wellness plan. Our goal is not to increase DHEA levels to multiple times their physiologic levels; rather, our goal is to keep them at an optimum level that maximizes your health and vitality.

Some laboratories also evaluate salivary samples of DHEA. You will need to refer to the documentation provided from the particular lab to fully evaluate this type of DHEA testing.

Laboratories may report DHEA and DHEA-S reference values based on age group. The following tables from *Dynacare Laboratories' Reference Manual* illustrate this method for free (unbound) DHEA and DHEA-S.

As you can see, the "normal" reference values for DHEA-S levels can be quite low and still be interpreted by the laboratory as normal, in no need of supplementation. However, I have found in clinical practice that the lower levels—especially less than 100 mcg/dl—are indeed associated with greater stress symptoms and respond well to supplemental pharmaceutical grade DHEA.

TABLE 5.1

DHEA Free, or Unbound (Active Form) via Blood Sample

UNITS OF MEASURE		EXCELLENT	GOOD	FAIR	LOW	SERIOUS DEFICIENCY
ng/dl	Men	750–1250	600–749	350–599	180–349	Less than 180
	Women	550–980	450–549	300–449	130–299	Less than 130

TABLE 5.2

DHEA-S, or Sulfated DHEA (Storage Form) via Blood Sample

UNITS OF MEASURE		EXCELLENT	GOOD	LOW	SERIOUS DEFICIENCY
mcg/dl	Men	450–600	300–450	125–300	Less than 125
	Women	280–380	150–280	45–150	Less than 45

TABLE 5.3

DHEA Laboratory Reference Values Based on Age and Sex (in ng/dl)

1–5 years	25–170 ng/dl
6–7 years	25–360 ng/dl
8–10 years	40–450 ng/dl
11–18 years	210–1,105 ng/dl**

**Levels vary according to sexual development

Males > 18 years	210–1,040 ng/dl
Females 19–50 years	210–1,040 ng/dl
Females > 50 years	70–210 ng/dl

DHEA depletion may be simply due to biology—a woman's body may have stopped producing DHEA in all but minute quantities. More likely, a low level is caused by stressful living. Whatever the cause, DHEA depletion leads directly to a lessening of patience and coping ability until, eventually, everything and everyone gets on our nerves. Impatience and frustration then give rise to negative changes in behavior and lifestyle.

As indicated below, very low levels of DHEA are also associated with exhaustion and serious illness.

Maintaining adequate levels of DHEA allows the body to adapt to life

TABLE 5.4

**DHEA-S Laboratory Reference Values
Based on Age and Sex (in mcg/dl)**

AGE	MALE	FEMALE
< 20 years	—no normals listed—	
20–29 years	102–597 mcg/dl	62–615 mcg/dl
30–39 years	109–666 mcg/dl	52–400 mcg/dl
40–49 years	50–517 mcg/dl	44–352 mcg/dl
50–59 years	63–444 mcg/dl	39–183 mcg/dl
> 59 years	32–154 mcg/dl	11–150 mcg/dl

TABLE 5.5

Relation of DHEA Level to Body State

DHEA LEVEL	BODY STATE
Excellent	Homeostasis (normal healthy function)
Good	Adaptation
Fair	Maladaptation
Low	Degeneration
Serious	Exhaustion and serious illness

stressors with vigor and vitality. Lifestyle modification, including supplementation with high-quality DHEA, can play a major additional role in returning DHEA levels to a safe range and keeping them there.

DHEA and Disease

In chapter 2 we discussed the fact that increased stress was associated with increased risk for many diseases. Numerous studies show a correlation between several disease states and a low DHEA-S level. Since DHEA acts in so many places in the body it is no surprise that a lack of DHEA or a significant depletion of DHEA could also have a profound effect on multiple organ systems in the body. Simply put, DHEA appears to be very protective, and the lack of this important hormone sets us up for a multitude of health-related problems.

DHEA and the Brain

The levels of DHEA in the brain are up to 6.5 times higher than DHEA levels found in other tissues of the body. This finding was reported by E. R. Braverman, M.D., in the February 1994 issue of *Total Health*. Brain neurons and the associated neurotransmitters are intimately involved in our behavior and our activity. It is to our benefit to protect this all-important communication system that governs who we are and what we do. Dopamine, a key neurotransmitter responsible for motivation, creativity, and general feelings of wellness, is an example of one such brain chemical that needs protection. The January 2003 issue of the journal *Synapse* emphasized the positive effects of DHEA in offering protection to dopamine neurons, which support an elevated mood.

DHEA and Depression

Depression, a common illness in our nation, is usually treated with prescription antidepressants. A study published in the journal *Psychopharmacology* in May 2002 confirmed that DHEA "is associated with an improvement in the symptoms of depression." In a related study performed the same year, researchers in the divisions of Young Adult Medicine and Endocrinology at Children's Hospital in Boston reported that in 61 women DHEA resulted in improvements in "specific psychological parameters." These positive results were similar to those found when DHEA was tested in the elderly population. Further studies relating a positive benefit from DHEA on mood were described in the journal *Trends in Endocrinology and Metabolism* in March 2002, where researchers claimed that DHEA acts as a neurosteroid (steroidlike molecule acting on the nervous system) on various neurotransmitter receptors (for example, dopamine and serotonin) in the brain. A decrease in the neurotransmitter serotonin is directly related to depressive symptoms and increased anxiety. The research highlighted the beneficial positive effects on mood, well-being, and sexuality in patients who suffered from adrenal insufficiency or mood disorders.

In my practice I have effectively used DHEA for many patients with symptoms of depression and anxiety. Their response is rapid, and due to its minimal side-effect profile, it has been a good first-line treatment for many patients with this condition.

DHEA and Osteoporosis

In their November 2002 issue the *Journal of Clinical Endocrinology and Metabolism* reported that both DHEA and hormone replacement therapy [HRT—estrogen and progesterone] "significantly reduced levels of certain bone resorption (bone-thinning) markers," indicating that both DHEA and HRT decreased the risk for osteoporosis.

DHEA and Diabetes

The Diabetes Endocrinology Research Center at the Veterans Affairs Medical Center, University of Iowa, published research supporting the positive effects of DHEA on vascular and neural function. They hypothesized that the positive benefits seen in their patients have been from the ability of DHEA to prevent oxidative stress (degeneration of tissues from oxygen-related free radicals), leading to improvement in both the circulation and the nerve problems that plague diabetic patients. Researchers at the Department of Experimental Medicine and Oncology at the University of Turin (Italy) published research raising the possibility that DHEA may protect the brain from diabetes-dependent damage.

DHEA and Cancer

DHEA has also been promoted as having benefit in warding off certain types of cancer. A promising study from the Third Department of Internal Medicine, Yokohama City University School of Medicine in Kanagawa, Japan, suggests that DHEA might be a potential chemoprotective agent against colon cancer.

DHEA and Cortisol

Cortisol levels increase with stress and are sustained at high levels when stress is constant. A study appearing in the French journal *Encéphale* (2002) reviewed the intimate relationship between DHEA and cortisol. The French researchers confirmed that persistent stress leads to an increased and prolonged biological level of cortisol. Elevated cortisol levels over an extended time are associated with increased psychological distress and a sense of loss of control. It is interesting and predictable that these are precisely the symptoms that hundreds of my patients relate to me in my office.

In this study researchers clarified the antistress role of DHEA. They considered that DHEA combated the negative effects of sustained elevated cortisol levels by acting as an antagonist to cortisol. Their findings confirmed that DHEA opposes the action of cortisol by "exerting a true anti-cortisol effect." They found that high cortisol levels were associated with a high level of anxiety, rumination (excessive worried thinking and recurrent thoughts), and negative attitude. This was seen much less frequently in patients with elevated DHEA-S levels.

These findings support the promise of The Stress Cure: In order to avert the biological effects of stress (elevated cortisol), we must increase levels of the "antidote" by increasing the body's level of DHEA. Decreased anxiety, improved mood, fewer feelings of being overwhelmed, and improved coping ability are only a few of the changes patients report soon after beginning natural DHEA supplementation.

DHEA Alone

To Kate it seemed as though stress had gotten the best of her overnight. One day everything was fine. The next day her life seemed to be a wreck. She had an argument with a coworker, and suddenly she hated her job. When her husband wasn't sympathetic enough, she blew up at him and their relationship took a turn for the worse. She felt "unnaturally jittery," she said, but blamed it on her kids, who always seemed to want something from her. Then she had trouble sleeping, which made her eat more. This made exercise more difficult, so she stopped, which caused her to gain even more weight and become self-conscious. None of these developments helped her mood, which became more anxious and irritable.

Kate had been my patient for several years, so I was surprised to see her looking so harried when she came in to see me. Worry lines crossed her forehead, and her usual hearty glow was gone.

"What's up?" I asked, sitting across from her.

She told me her story, all the while looking puzzled.

"The strange thing to me is that everything I told you is normal in my life," she said. "Fights with my coworkers aren't uncommon, and I don't always get along with my husband. My kids always want something from me. The difference was the way I responded. It was like a switch had been thrown, and I suddenly went batty."

I explained the premise of female stress to her and how the gradual reduction of DHEA in a woman's body can lead to unusual reactions to usual events.

Not wanting her condition to worsen, Kate began to take DHEA in the amounts that I will describe in this chapter. Using DHEA alone, Kate's mood improved dramatically. As her DHEA levels climbed to healthy levels, her weight began to drop and her robust skin color returned.

Kate felt better than she had in months, she told me during a follow-up visit. She would eventually go on to implement much of the other advice in this book—stress reduction, diet improvement, supplements, sleep, and repairing relationships—but even just taking DHEA had lowered the stress level in her life.

DHEA alone can do that. Study after study confirms what I see on a daily basis among my patients: DHEA alone can reduce female stress significantly.

Getting Started

Your next questions might be:

- "How do I know if my DHEA levels are low?"
- "How do I take DHEA?"
- "If 25 mg per day of DHEA is good, why isn't 400 mg better?"
- "How do I talk to my doctor about taking DHEA?"

These are good questions because they illustrate the careful thinking you should do before taking any kind of medication or following any health plan, including The Stress Cure.

Before you start taking any pills, I am going to explain how to start, take, and monitor your intake of DHEA. I will also help guide you in discussing this option with your doctor. The point of this chapter is not only to help raise your DHEA levels but also to assist your doctor in understanding what female stress is, what causes it, and how he or she can help you improve your health status and reverse its detrimental effects.

By requesting DHEA, you are asking for something that is out of the ordinary for many physicians. Be patient when presenting this information to your doctor, but be firm as well. Explain that there are many ways to deal with the constellation of symptoms known as female stress and that you want to try the most natural method you can find.

Many medical doctors are changing to a more holistic approach to medicine, largely because of pressure from patients who are becoming increasingly cautious about the side effects of modern medications. There is also a movement by baby boomers to take more control of their health care, reminding me of the words of the Chinese poet Lao-tzu, who wrote: "My life is in my hands, not in the control of heaven and earth."

Doctor Talk: Communicating Medical Style

Let us assume that you have access to a health care practitioner who is willing to work with you to get to the bottom of why you are feeling poorly. Your first step may be a thorough medical examination. You may find it helpful to follow the outline below in preparing for the office visit with your doctor. Take time to write out the answers to these questions so that your physician can use this information to help formulate a plan to begin to reverse the detrimental effects of stress.

The Medical History

Start by writing down exactly how you are feeling. Just let the words flow. Then review what you have written and highlight the items of most significance to you. Do this before you go to the doctor's office.

Once you have developed a general statement about the state of your health, it is time to create a detailed medical history, which your doctor will need in order to be able to provide a complete evaluation.

Chief Complaint

List your primary complaint right up front. This is called the chief complaint or primary complaint. What is the main reason for your visit to the doctor? Have you come because of weight concerns? Depression? Anxiety? Fatigue? All of the above? This gives the doctor an indication of the main problem that needs to be addressed.

Present the Problem

This is where you get to tell your story about the sleepless nights, the inability to function, the fatigue, the feelings of despair and sadness, and so on. Or talk about the anger and rage, the inability to control your feelings, the yelling, and the headaches. This is your opportunity to really tell it like it is. Describe everything you are experiencing. Hold nothing back.

Medications

Which medications are you taking? List all of the prescription and nonprescription drugs, therapeutic supplements, vitamins, and minerals you are taking. Don't forget to include medications such as aspirin or Tylenol and birth control pills.

Allergies

List any and all prescription and nonprescription medications you are allergic to, and describe what happened when you had a reaction.

Medical History

List all the major illnesses you have had in the past, any complications you may have had, and the outcomes. Were you hospitalized? If so, for how long? Where? Have any residual problems persisted after the illness?

Do you have any ongoing chronic medical conditions? Are there specific treatments you are currently undergoing? Which specialists, if any, are caring for you?

Past Surgical History

List all surgeries and their approximate dates. Include any complications, special circumstances, or problems associated with the surgeries or in the postoperative periods.

Social History

Where are you currently living and with whom? Who makes up your family? Are there any problems, concerns, or frustrations at home? How are your finances? Who shares in the household chores and responsibilities?

Review of Symptoms

Now it is time for you to talk about the gritty details related to the various physical, psychological, and other concerns you are currently experiencing. This review will allow your health care provider to get a complete sense of your problem. Remember that you and your doctor are putting together a complex picture of many interacting organ systems.

To save time and make sure you have covered all of your symptoms, you may choose to use the Medical Symptoms Questionnaire below. It covers some of the areas that I feel are important to identify. Note: Make certain to include symptoms that you have "learned to live with."

MEDICAL SYMPTOMS
QUESTIONNAIRE (reprinted with permission of Immuno Laboratory, Inc.)

Digestive Tract
- ❑ Diarrhea
- ❑ Constipation
- ❑ Bloated feeling
- ❑ Belching
- ❑ Passing gas
- ❑ Stomach pains

Ears
- ❑ Itchy ears
- ❑ Ear aches
- ❑ Ear infections
- ❑ Drainage from ears
- ❑ Ringing in ears
- ❑ Hearing loss

Emotions
- ❑ Mood swings
- ❑ Anxiety, fear
- ❑ Irritability, anger
- ❑ Depression
- ❑ Aggressiveness
- ❑ Nervousness

Energy & Activity
- ❑ Fatigue
- ❑ Sluggishness
- ❑ Apathy
- ❑ Hyperactivity
- ❑ Restlessness
- ❑ Lethargy

Eyes
- ❑ Watery eyes
- ❑ Itchy eyes
- ❑ Swollen eyelids
- ❑ Dark circles
- ❑ Blurred vision

Weight
- ❑ Binge eating
- ❑ Cravings
- ❑ Excessive weight
- ❑ Compulsive eating
- ❑ Water retention
- ❑ Underweight

Joint & Muscles
- ❑ Pain in joints
- ❑ Arthritis
- ❑ Stiffness
- ❑ Limited movement
- ❑ Aches in muscles
- ❑ Feeling of weakness

Mouth & Throat
- ❑ Chronic coughing
- ❑ Gagging
- ❑ Often clear throat
- ❑ Sore throat
- ❑ Swollen tongue/lips
- ❑ Canker sores

Nose
- ❑ Stuffy nose
- ❑ Sinus problems
- ❑ Hay fever
- ❑ Sneezing attacks
- ❑ Excessive mucous

Head
- ❑ Headaches
- ❑ Faintness
- ❑ Dizziness
- ❑ Insomnia

Skin
- ❑ Acne
- ❑ Hives, rashes
- ❑ Hair loss
- ❑ Flushing/hot flashes
- ❑ Excessive sweating

Lungs
- ❑ Chest congestion
- ❑ Asthma, bronchitis
- ❑ Shortness of breath
- ❑ Difficulty breathing

Mind
- ❑ Poor memory
- ❑ Confusion
- ❑ Poor concentration
- ❑ Stuttering/ stammering
- ❑ Learning disabilities

Other
- ❑ Irregular heartbeat
- ❑ Rapid heartbeat
- ❑ Chest pains
- ❑ Frequent illness
- ❑ Urgent urination
- ❑ Genital itch

General Physical Exam

A general physical examination may be recommended or performed if you request it, if something in your history or presentation of symptoms suggests that a physical exam is necessary, or if your doctor feels it is indicated. Your doctor will examine your chest, heart, and abdomen for signs of physical disease. A musculoskeletal exam and limited neurological examination will probably also be performed. Particular attention should be paid to the sinuses, neck, and thyroid. A breast exam with a mammogram and a Pap smear and pelvic exam should be performed per recommended guidelines if indicated. Additional studies such as a chest X ray, EKG (electrocardiogram), and bone density test also may be necessary.

Laboratory Examinations

Several laboratory studies are recommended for those patients suffering from symptoms that are fueled by stress. A general blood evaluation, called a CBC, or complete blood count, evaluates white cells (which fight infections), red cells (which carry oxygen), and platelets (which help your blood clot). A general chemistry panel is useful for checking glucose, liver enzymes, kidney function, protein levels, gallbladder, and electrolytes such as sodium, potassium, and chloride. Total cholesterol and both "good" (HDL) and "bad" (LDL) cholesterol should be evaluated, along with triglycerides. Calcium and phosphorus may be tested, as well as thyroid hormones. In patients who are overweight I frequently screen for diabetes by testing for fructosamine, hemoglobin A1c, and serum insulin. Levels of the hormones estrogen, progesterone, testosterone, and DHEA are also tested (along with FSH and LH if indicated). I also recommend testing C-reactive protein and homocysteine levels in many patients, as elevations in these levels can be associated with an increased risk for atherosclerosis and heart-related health problems.

Other laboratory testing is ordered depending on individual indications or as a result of findings obtained during the physical examination or medical history. Most of the lab results are returned within a few days, when patients return for a face-to-face follow-up discussion.

Assessment and Plan

Bringing all of this information together and drawing conclusions is the art of medical doctors and health care providers. The goal is first to recognize the patterns of symptoms and stress-related disease, and then to create and implement workable and logical solutions to maximize your health.

I frequently prepare a co-morbidity list of all the interrelated problems, so as to keep an eye on the forest and not just the individual trees. After developing this list, I meet with the patient to develop a logical plan to complete further diagnostic tests and to implement therapeutic interventions.

It is critical that you be involved in this process with your physician. If your doctor tells you to do something you know you just won't do, you will set yourself up for failure (and noncompliance in the eyes of your doctor). I frequently ask my patients what they are *able* to do and what they *will* do. Will they walk five minutes a day this week? Will they decrease their cigarette smoking by one cigarette per week? Can they afford the nutritional supplements that are recommended? Will they take them? All of these things need to be taken into consideration when outlining a treatment plan.

Remember that it is not good enough to bring you from sick to not sick. We must continue to get you to well and then to very well.

Testing: Are Your DHEA Levels Too Low?

As I mentioned at the beginning of this chapter, your DHEA levels can be tested through your serum (blood) or saliva.

With the serum method, a tube of blood is drawn from a vein in your arm and sent to a laboratory for analysis. I prefer this method because it can measure either free DHEA or the storage, or sulfated, form called DHEA-S. We currently use Labcorp for our DHEA-S blood testing. The cost of the test is low, and they have laboratory locations in thousands of cities across the United States. For more information about obtaining a blood DHEA-S test, please see the reference section or go online at www.thestresscure.com.

Some clinicians prefer saliva testing, but the levels in saliva are less stable even though they identify the true state of the free, or active, hormone. I have many patients who prefer saliva tests because they can be conducted at home and then mailed to the lab for analysis. When we test with saliva, we use the Great Smokies Diagnostic Laboratory, which performs testing for several hormones, including DHEA and cortisol, called the Adrenal Stress Profile. The cost of the test varies depending on what is being evaluated and may include nutritional recommendations or suggestions, but it does not take the place of a professional evaluation and diagnosis from a health care provider. If you have any problems obtaining saliva testing of your DHEA level, you may call or write our office to request a Saliva DHEA/Cortisol Test Kit. You may also obtain more information and order kits from the www.thestresscure.com Web site.

Taking DHEA: Less Is More

I recommend starting DHEA supplementation when DHEA-S levels fall below 60 mcg/dl in women and below 100 mcg/dl in men. I also recommend supplementing with DHEA if patients have slightly higher DHEA-S levels and have many of the stress-associated symptoms discussed in this book. DHEA supplementation is then increased as necessary to raise DHEA-S blood levels to a more respectable level of 150–280 mcg/dl in women and 300–450 mcg/dl in men. Excellent levels would be in the 280–360 mcg/dl for females and 450–600 mcg/dl for males.

How Is This Done?

A good rule of thumb with DHEA is Less is more. This can be interpreted two ways. First, you want to take only the amount of DHEA necessary to restore your levels to a more healthy state. There is no added value in having DHEA levels that are sky-high, and there may be added harm in taking amounts that are far greater than needed.

In following that rule, I usually start my female patients on 25 mg per day of supplemental, pure DHEA (98% or higher) if testing shows that their DHEA-S levels are below 60 mcg/dl. If a patient is sensitive to medications or has had trouble tolerating any stimulants or supplements in the past, I will begin at only 5–10 mg per day. If she has high blood pressure or any heart disease, I usually proceed more cautiously, with 5–10 mg per day as the initial dose.

Who Should *Not* Take DHEA?

DHEA is not for everyone. For example, children should not take DHEA. Neither should women who are pregnant, lactating, or planning to become pregnant. You should also avoid DHEA if you are on hormone therapy (including estrogen, oral contraceptive agents, or corticosteroids), have a hyperandrogenic condition, or have breast, uterine, or ovarian cancer.

DHEA is *not* indicated if there is any history of breast cancer, for men if they have prostate cancer, or any estrogen- or testosterone-related tumor.

Since DHEA is converted by the body into the active sex hormones estrogen and testosterone, anyone with a medical condition that could be negatively affected by increased sex hormones in the body should avoid taking DHEA without the advice of her health care provider. I always encourage patients to seek the advice and cooperation of a health care professional with expertise and experience in using DHEA. Some doctors will not recommend taking DHEA under any circumstances because they may not understand its positive effects. I caution physicians not to make this error with their patients. If a health care provider is not familiar with DHEA supplementation or lacks the expertise to evaluate a patient with respect to DHEA, it is best just to admit that and refer the patient elsewhere.

What Dosage Is Best?

The most frequent dosage level of DHEA I give to my patients is 25–50 mg per day. The next most common level is 10 mg three times per day, especially for those women who take the necessary steps to reduce their stress levels by following recommendations discussed in steps 2–7 of The Stress Cure.

If a patient has trouble sleeping, I advise her to take the full DHEA dose in the morning, since taking DHEA in the evening can potentially interfere with sleep. This problem has occurred in only a fraction of my patients. Most take DHEA twice daily: in the morning and later in the afternoon. At either the 25 mg or 50 mg level, patients have had few side effects and an excellent therapeutic response. It is rare that I need to increase the dosage higher than 50 mg, and I do so only after reviewing DHEA laboratory results six weeks after initial treatment.

Visible Results

When my female patients are feeling their worst, their DHEA levels have been at their lowest. As the levels rise after we begin supplementation, these women experience positive changes in behavior, attitude, energy, and function, and they feel better than they have in months or even years. Much of the literature states that the effects of DHEA supplementation can take months to appear, but my patients have experienced quite the opposite— sometimes feeling the effects of DHEA supplementation in just a few days. In fact, some patients have said that they have begun to feel better within hours.

Here are some examples of patients who have had rapid improvement with just the use of DHEA:

Andrea: From 32 mcg/dL to 403 mcg/dl   Calling herself "an emotional washout," Andrea's DHEA-S blood level was only 32 mcg/dl. After taking 25 mg per day for a week, then increasing to 50 mg per day of DHEA for two months, Andrea felt "like a rocket," she said, because she was "spewing good humor" almost all of the time.

Kara: From zero to 379 mcg/dl   "It was like going from black and white to Technicolor," said Kara. Her DHEA-S blood level was zero! I started her on 50 mg per day of DHEA (since her level was undetectable), and she responded very quickly, her levels rising until they reached a high of 379 mcg/dl after four months of supplementation. "It was great to see the world as I did when I was in my twenties and thirties," she said.

Sally: From 23 mcg/dl to 410 mcg/dl   "This must be what it feels like to discover the fountain of youth," said Sally, who had been severely blue for several years before starting DHEA supplementation. I put her on 25 mg per day for the first week, then increased her to 50 mg per day of DHEA, and then gradually had her start the other aspects of the program, such as exercise, diet, and stress reduction. Sally responded quickly, her DHEA-S level climbing to 410 mcg/dl in only two months. "As my levels went up, so did my mood," said Sally. "It was like turning up the volume on my body's energy system."

Jenn: From 44 mcg/dl to 380 mcg/dl   "I was unhappy all the time and I didn't know why," said Jenn. "I was distant from my coworkers, and always stressed and angry when someone came into my office to talk. I just didn't want human contact." Her DHEA-S level was 44 mcg/dl. A little over three months later she was referring to herself as the"new Jenn." As she put it: "DHEA is a mood-altering substance, and I am glad of it."

These are just a few of the hundreds of examples from my practice. These four, however, clearly make the case: DHEA alone can change nighttime into day when it comes to female stress.

Take the Best

Due to its profound influence throughout the body, I recommend that my patients take only the highest-quality DHEA they can find. I have found that DHEA supplements made with calcium carbonate do not seem to be as effective. It may be that the calcium carbonate interferes with absorption or some other factor, but many patients find a clear difference when taking a pure DHEA supplement without the calcium carbonate added. This is one supplement I do not recommend buying off the discount shelf. I cannot underscore enough the benefit of knowing where your supplements come from and trusting the source for any supplements you take, especially DHEA. Look in appendix section of this book for a list of recommended DHEA supplements that we have found from reputable manufacturers.

As with other supplements, the manufacture of DHEA is not regulated by the federal Food and Drug Administration, so its safety and efficacy are not closely monitored. A letter published in the *Journal of the American Medical Association (JAMA)* seriously called into question self-prescribing DHEA based in part on the lack of standardization in some supplements. The authors examined 16 randomly selected products in the laboratory. Only seven of those were found to have the DHEA content within the typical pharmaceutical product specifications of 90–110% of the labeled claim. Of the others, one product contained no DHEA, and two contained only trace amounts. Two others claimed that they contained naturally occurring DHEA (an unlikely promise, since DHEA is manufactured by the adrenal glands and is not found in other so-called natural sources such as plants, water, or animal products). Yet another contained 150% of the labeled amount of DHEA.

The take-home message here: Buyer beware. Read labels carefully and use only brands of DHEA and other supplements whose reliability and manufacturing processes are trustworthy. It is also recommended that you consult your personal physician or health care provider for assistance in finding a good source for DHEA and other natural supplements.

My Recommendation

One of the forms of DHEA that we recommend in our Seattle clinic is obtained from PhysioLogics. The DHEA sold by PhysioLogics is derived from diosgenin, a substance extracted from natural sources and then converted into DHEA. PhysioLogics guarantees that their DHEA is 98.5% pure. I have personally inspected the manufacturing facilities of Physio-Logics and found them to be of the highest caliber.

Another source of DHEA that we utilize is from Douglas Laboratories. Douglas Labs has been a leader in the field of physician-recommended nutritional supplements, and their quality has been impressive.

Metagenics is another company that we utilize frequently for many of our nutritional products. Metagenics has a state-of-the-art manufacturing facility that I have visited, located in Gig Harbor, Washington. Metagenics works closely with health care providers and has one of the best physician educational series in the industry.

Our medical wellness company, Health*Max*, has several forms of high-quality DHEA available on its Web site at www.healthmax.net or by calling 206-362-1111. The Web site www.thestresscure.com is also a source for obtaining high-quality DHEA. Both sites provide the option to order online.

Many of our patients prefer sublingual forms of DHEA—the type that dissolves under the tongue. One brand that we recommend to our patients is produced by Douglas Laboratories. Sublingual forms can be found in many health stores across the country and are high-quality nutritional supplements.

Special Forms of DHEA

There are specialized forms of DHEA available, and they can be of benefit in some specific situations. Below you will find the various forms and a description of the benefits of each:

- ### DHEA Liposomal Spray

This form of DHEA usually comes in bottles that deliver 2–5 mg of DHEA per spray. Liposomal DHEA, which is sprayed under the tongue, delivers the nutrient quickly, is rapidly absorbed by the oral mucosa, and maintains a sustained effect over an extended period of time. The liposomal spray form is particularly beneficial for those who may have difficulty absorbing nutrients or swallowing tablets or capsules. Each manufacturer's spray has its own unique flavor.

Liposomal DHEA is found with greater than 99.8% purity, exceeding pharmaceutical standards for purity. A common dose would be one to five sprays under the tongue daily, holding for 20 seconds and then swallowing. Both Metagenics and PhysioLogics sell liposomal forms of DHEA.

- ### 7-keto DHEA

The technical name for this compound is 3-beta-acetoxyarost-5-en-7 17 dione. It is much easier, however, to say 7-keto DEHA. The compound 7-keto DHEA does not metabolize to form testosterone or estrogen like the common form of DHEA supplements, so you do not have to worry about its impact on sex hormones. Like DHEA, 7-keto DHEA is formed naturally within the body. Taking 7-keto DHEA avoids the potential risk of the possible cancer-promoting effects of certain forms of estrogen.

A dilemma that is faced by patients with a history of breast cancer and their doctors is whether or not to use supplemental DHEA. Since DHEA converts to estrogen, I do *not* recommend that breast cancer survivors take supplemental DHEA, but I do recommend that they follow the other six steps of the de-Stress program. Patients who are at high risk for estrogen-influenced cancers should also refrain from the regular form of DHEA. The 7-keto form may be a logical alternative for this population, since it provides the benefits of DHEA without the negative effect of increasing estrogen. I strongly urge any woman who is at risk for breast disease or who has had confirmed breast cancer to work closely with her oncologist before taking any DHEA-related supplement.

DHEA may be beneficial preventively, as research suggests that low levels of DHEA are associated with an increased risk for breast cancer, especially in younger women. For this reason we advocate testing DHEA levels early and supplementing with DHEA to maintain normal physiologic levels. If your testosterone level is already elevated or normal, you can take 7-keto DHEA without fear of causing it to rise any further. Other estrogen- or testosterone-related conditions, such as acne, may also be prevented by 7-keto DHEA. Since this form of DHEA does not elevate testosterone, it is also helpful for those concerned about excessive hair growth.

Animal and in vitro studies indicate that 7-keto DHEA is more potent than DHEA for enhancing the immune system (by increasing interleukin-2 levels in the blood) and improving memory retention. 7-keto DHEA has undergone rigorous toxicology assessments and has been evaluated for safety in double-blind, placebo-controlled clinical research trials.

7-keto DHEA has also been evaluated for use in weight loss. In one study, participants were given either 100 mg of 7-keto DHEA or a placebo. All subjects were put on an 1,800 calorie-per-day diet and advised to exercise for 45 minutes, three times per week. After eight weeks individuals taking the 7-keto DHEA had lost an average of 6.34 pounds, compared with a 2.13-pound loss for the group that had taken the placebo. The weight loss was attributable to an increase in the thyroid hormone.T_3, but levels did not exceed the normal range.

• Sublingual DHEA 5 mg and 25 mg
Sublingual DHEA is formulated to be placed under the tongue and allowed to dissolve slowly. This pleasant-tasting form is an excellent choice for those

patients who do not wish to swallow tablets or pills. Some nutritionists believe that as the sublingual tablet dissolves, the active ingredient is absorbed readily by the highly vascular area under the tongue. It is then taken up directly by the bloodstream, avoiding any degradation by the liver, which occurs when supplements are absorbed from the stomach or intestines. Others think that even though sublingual forms dissolve under the tongue, most of the active ingredient is actually swallowed and absorbed via the normal route.

- ## Compounded DHEA Cream

DHEA can also be compounded into a smooth cream that is absorbed into the bloodstream when applied to a highly vascular area like the lower wrist. A physician will need to order this for you. Compounding pharmacists can make up the cream, which contains a specific amount per 1/10th of a milliliter of cream, about the size of a small pea. This is easily rubbed on the skin, and the active ingredient is absorbed without passing through the stomach or liver.

- ## Specialty Formulations: Stress*Free*

Sometimes you will find DHEA combined with other compounds designed to work in concert for a given purpose. As an example, a product I designed and formulated for my patients is called Stress*Free*. Stress-*Free* was designed especially for those patients complaining of lethargy and fatigue in addition to their stress. It may also help those feeling down and blue from periods of prolonged stress. Each tablet contains 10 mg of DHEA. It should be taken two or three times a day to obtain a 20–30 mg daily dose of DHEA. In addition to DHEA, the following nutrients have been added to the formulation:

- **Tyrosine**   An essential amino acid with demonstrated ability to help the brain cope with stress. Tyrosine is utilized in the production of norepinephrine (an energy hormone) and dopamine, another key neurotransmitter. Both norepinephrine and dopamine play active roles in our behavior and our overall feelings of well-being. Studies have indicated that tyrosine supplementation can lift mood, increase attentiveness, and enhance sexual desire.
- **Vitamin B$_{12}$ (cobalamin)**   Important for the proper functioning of the immune system, nerves, and energy metabolism, cobalamin helps to energize both the body and the brain. This impor-

tant vitamin is used to combat depression, Alzheimer's disease, and asthma, as well as mental disorders resulting from prolonged B_{12} deficiency.

- **Ginseng**   This compound has been shown to enhance memory and physical capabilities. One of the world's most popular herbs, ginseng is commonly used to fight stress and increase vitality.
- **Vitamin B₅ (pantothenic acid)**   Vital for the adrenal glands, pantothenic acid aids in the production of adrenal hormones and red blood cells. It also stimulates the immune system, boosts energy levels, and has a positive influence on the way a body utilizes fats and carbohydrates. Studies have shown that pantothenic acid plays an important role in arming the body against stress.
- **Saint-John's-wort**   Proven effective in treating mild to moderate depression without the side effects of standard antidepressants. Saint-John's-wort also protects against infections and is used in the treatment of chronic, stress-related insomnia and anxiety. Saint-John's-wort was added to StressFree to promote the activity of serotonin, a neurotransmitter that plays an important role in mood elevation.
- **Zinc**   The numerous enzymes in this mineral play important roles in protein synthesis, supporting the immune system, speeding the body's healing process, and helping the mind stay alert. Zinc is involved in maintaining healthy skin and the nervous, digestive, and reproductive systems. Experts believe that most Americans do not have sufficient zinc in their diet; up to 75% of the country's population falls short of recommended zinc levels.
- **DHEA Plus**   DHEA Plus is a combination supplement containing 25 mg of DHEA and 25 mg of pregnenolone. Pregnenolone, a metabolite of cholesterol, is the precursor to both DHEA and cortisol. In some patients with prolonged stress levels, cortisol can become depleted similar to DHEA. Adding small amounts of pregnenolone can assist the body in normalizing cortisol levels. Caution should be used when taking pregnenolone. It has been reported that taking excessive pregnenolone has been associated with abnormal heart rhythms in some patients.

Side Effects

Caution is again underscored here. Use these supplements with a great deal of respect. They are potent hormones and prohormones and can have a significant beneficial effect when taken in an appropriate dose to restore your DHEA levels to a more healthy value.

Although side effects are rare and usually associated only with excessive doses of DHEA, they can include hair loss, increased facial hair, acne, menstrual irregularities, irritability, restlessness, and heart palpitations and/or irregularities. Acne can be an annoying side effect that may occur even at small doses of DHEA. Some patients report that the acne is short-lived, and they continue taking DHEA without further symptoms. Other patients discontinue the supplement in favor of 7-keto DHEA, which usually avoids this nuisance. Although I have never had a patient with cardiac symptoms from DHEA, as with any supplement or prescription, if you experience any side effects, stop the DHEA and consult your health care provider.

The Miracle Hormone?

As I have stated several times in this book, my patients consistently and predictably experience profound improvement with DHEA. Patients from all walks of life report feeling better—within days—after beginning this natural nutritional supplement. Having written my fair share of prescription medications to treat depression and anxiety in the past, I now rarely have to prescribe these therapeutic agents. Many of my patients are able to effectively discontinue their prescription antidepressant or antianxiety medications and are able to feel much better, with fewer side effects, naturally.

But DHEA alone is not the answer. It is not a one-size-fits-all treatment. DHEA is a major component in the comprehensive antistress (De-STRESS) program discussed in the chapters that follow. *With* DHEA as the first step, steps 2–7 will be easier to implement. *Without* DHEA, you may have the right goals and the best of intentions, but judging from what I see in my practice, it will probably be difficult for you to accomplish what you set out to achieve.

Think of DHEA as the wind beneath the wings of motivational change and behavioral improvement. Without it, you stay on the ground. With it, you have unlimited potential to lift your spirit and you health!

CHAPTER SIX

Step 2: Supplemental Nutrition

Only recently have vitamins begun to receive the respect they deserve from the medical community. In the past some medical doctors even went so far as to describe the only benefit of vitamin supplements as giving the patient "expensive urine."

In the past few years vitamins and various nutritional supplements have been shown to do far more than simply make for expensive urine. This is especially true in the area of stress control. Prolonged and excessive stress—whether due to emotional, environmental, or physical causes—depletes key nutrients needed to renew the body's stress-fighting factors. Vitamin supplements can help replace those nutrients.

In this chapter I am going to explain why you may need supplements, even if you eat a healthy, nutritious diet. I will describe many different vitamins, explain their functions within your body, tell you where they can be found naturally in foods, and give you guidelines for safe supplementation. At the end of the chapter I will discuss some specific vitamin and supplement formulas that I routinely recommend to my patients.

The History of Molecular Nutrition

These days it seems we are awash in a tidal wave of information about vitamins, minerals, herbs, and nutritional supplements. As researchers expand their understanding of the actions, reactions, and interactions of food and its constituent parts, scientists are beginning to prove the long-held notion that vitamins are good for you.

Three icons get front-stage credit for bringing us to our current understanding about the relationship of food and nutrients to our health. In the 1950s Linus Pauling, Ph.D., opened our eyes to the field of research known as molecular medicine. He began to analyze what foodstuffs were made of at the molecular level and what nutrients our body needed to obtain from the foods we eat. Roger Williams, Ph.D., can be credited for developing the concept of biochemical individuality, the idea that each of us is uniquely different on a biochemical level far beyond our obvious differences in terms of facial features, eyes and hair color, and body type. Abram Hofer, M.D., Ph.D., introduced the concept of biomolecular psychiatry, relating certain behavioral and psychological states to imbalances in various molecular substances resulting from the intake of certain foods or from a lack of specific nutrients.

Let Food Be Our Medicine and Medicine Be Our Food

I have heard this saying many times over the years, but it didn't really stick with me until the mid-1990s. I attended a conference at the request of my friend and colleague Soheyla Mousavi, Ph.D. Dr. Mousavi is a soft-spoken, intelligent, and cheerful woman trained in clinical nutrition. She wanted me to come to listen to a talk given by Jeffrey Bland, Ph.D., whose mentor had been the Nobel laureate and vitamin C champion, Linus Pauling. "Soheyla, I must have it proven to me, beyond a shadow of a doubt, before I will start giving out vitamins to patients to cure their ills," I said, speaking from a 100% traditionally trained point of view. "I have heard stories about vitamins such as vitamin C helping people, and I'd like to believe them. But I need to see the data to be sure."

The conference I attended proved to be a turning point in my career. Not only did the data convince me, but the research was immense! How could my M.D. colleagues say, "There are no studies that support" this or that natural remedy, when a wealth of research studies existed about various natural treatments? I put on my student hat and began devouring everything I could get my hands on relating to food and its influence over health and "unhealth" or disease. I learned that our behavior, our stamina, our energy level, our ability to fight off infections—all were related *inti-*

mately to the food we eat. Wow! I felt like the geek who had missed the memo—and I began to reflect on my medical school training. During the years I was in medical school, we had about eight hours of training in nutrition, hardly time to provide more than an understanding of what a protein was and the difference between a fat and a carbohydrate. We also reviewed a few specialty diets created to help manage certain diseases. That was it! When I read the information from Dr. Bland and his cohorts, it was as if a light had been turned on in a very dark room.

I do not expect you to instantly develop the passion for this information that I did, but through this experience I realized that the information surrounding vitamins can be very confusing. Which are the right vitamins to take, what brands are considered top quality, and how much of them do we need to take? The answers were more difficult to find than I thought.

Nutritional Research

The term *vitamin* comes from the German word *vitamine,* which is a combination of two words: *vita*—meaning "life"—and *amine*—meaning an organic compound containing nitrogen. The word was first used by Polishborn American biochemist Casimir Funk in 1911. Since later study found that not all vitamins contained the nitrogen group, the *e* was dropped and *vitamin* has remained. The term is defined as a relatively complex organic substance that occurs in small amounts in animals and plants and is essential for the normal continuation of life functions.

With the increased interest today in alternative and natural methods of treatment, the National Institutes of Health (NIH) has been given millions of dollars to research the medical claims about various integrated treatments, such as vitamin supplements. The goal of the NIH is to distinguish products with false claims from those that provide actual therapeutic benefit.

We are fortunate to have some of the world's leaders in functional medicine and wellness-based health care here in the Northwest. Jeffrey Bland, along with his team of researchers at the Institute for Functional Medicine, has been in the forefront of this research for over 25 years. Jeff has been a key leader in functional medical education worldwide. Bastyr University has also been the home of Joe Pizzorno, N.D. (doctor of naturopathy), a highly regarded teacher of integrated medicine until his recent retirement from the university. Alan Gaby, M.D., Michael Murray, N.D.,

Jonathan Wright, M.D., and many other respected researchers also call the Northwest home, and they publish some of the world's best literature on the subject of wellness-based, or functional, medicine.

Germany is also at the forefront in evaluating alternative treatments and new discoveries in natural-functional medicine.

However, even with all this scientific information available, people often get much of their information on vitamins and supplements and other advances in health and wellness from tabloids and magazines. These sources are not always all bad, but the quality and accuracy of their information can be questionable and patients can be easily confused. The popular press is quick to jump on each new "discovery" or study result as a major breakthrough, and the public can be led to think that a small, initial finding that may have little clinical significance is the new gospel.

Developing a Reliable Source of Information

Along with some colleagues I decided to form a company called Health-*Max* to help patients learn about nutritional interventions and to help doctors learn about reputable sources of information regarding this "new" area of therapeutics. I felt this was necessary, since it was not obvious at first to me what products and which manufacturers were reputable and ethical. This is one reason why many physicians are very skeptical, and rightfully so, when it comes to recommending anything "natural." However, at a time when over 100,000 deaths occur each year from prescription medication taken at the correct dose, doctors are beginning at least to listen and look at the data on nutritional intervention. I believe it is physicians' responsibility to explore and learn about this useful segment of the health care industry in order to be able to offer comprehensive services to their patients. Patients are eager to discuss natural options with doctors who are willing to talk with them and not talk down to them or make them feel uneasy about asking for information.

HealthMax was created to help bridge the gap between traditional medical education and alternative or natural interventions—such as vitamin supplements—that may work as well as, or even better than, their prescription counterparts. You can visit our Web site to find additional information and to purchase vitamin supplements that you can be confident are of the highest quality. We also recommend reputable manufacturers in appendix section of this book.

The Power of Proper Nutrition

In its simplest form food is energy. As with your car, if you consume the right types and right amount of fuel, you go a long way toward peak performance and a long life. Skimp on the quality, quantity, or composition of the fuel and you run the risk of a breakdown or early demise.

No two women lead the same lives. Each woman is unique, and so are her nutritional and caloric needs. A blonde, blue-eyed, fine-boned woman of northern European descent who also happens to smoke is at risk for osteoporosis, so she may benefit from eating more foods containing calcium and vitamin D. An African-American woman who is not a smoker and whose risk of osteoporosis is inherently lower (because of her race and her larger frame) may be at a greater risk for high blood pressure. That risk should make her more conscious of keeping her sodium intake low and her consumption of heart-healthy vegetables high. Even with these distinctions, the operative word when it comes to nutrition remains balance. Without a balanced approach to personal nutrition, a woman is at risk of not having the essential vitamins, minerals, micronutrients, and calories she needs to stay healthy.

Marissa had never taken vitamins or any other nutritional supplements before I treated her for female stress syndrome. She said she didn't believe in them. She came to my office complaining of weight gain since the birth of her child three years earlier. Marissa, now 30 years old, had been trying in vain to lose weight. She ate less and less, but her weight continued to creep up. At five feet six inches, her ideal weight was around 130 pounds. Marissa had quit smoking years earlier and had remained a nonsmoker, for which I commended her greatly. "I have often thought about smoking again," she said. "It always made me lose weight in the past." She immediately dismissed this as an approach to help her shed the unwanted pounds, but she was quite frustrated that she had gained 52 pounds over her 130–135-pound baseline. Marissa, like many women I have cared for, felt constantly guilty about her weight. She was trying to diet by skipping meals and eating very little. She routinely skipped breakfast and only snacked for lunch. Dinner was usually centered around vegetables and fruit, but she had a hard time resisting the lure of carbohydrates. She had cut back on caffeine but didn't drink much water and drank three to four diet sodas daily. Despite all her activity chasing after a three-year-old, her weight didn't budge, causing her to overeat on occasion in frustration.

Marissa is an example of a roller-coaster eater. Eating too little, and then too much is always a challenge to the body. She was fatigued, felt achy in her muscles, had frequent headaches, and would experience occasional skipped heartbeats and dizziness throughout the week. Her dietary habits were severely depriving her body of the basics of good nutrition. She ate too many carbohydrates, too little quality protein, and went too long between meals. I needed to help Marissa understand the importance of providing her body with the essential vitamins, minerals, and trace elements that would help her return to being a healthy and vibrant young woman.

I recommended a saliva test for Marissa so that we could get an accurate assessment of her cortisol, DHEA, and testosterone levels. The testing kit came with four small vials to allow her to collect saliva four times over the next day and mail the samples to the lab. On the basis of her symptoms, it was clear that she would benefit from nutritional supplementation, and she scored poorly on the female stress questionnaire. Since she was experiencing so much stress, I felt comfortable with her beginning to take DHEA while we waited for the lab results on her saliva test. I recommended that she begin taking 25 mg of DHEA in the morning. In addition, I told her I wanted her to begin taking a high-potency multiple vitamin and mineral supplement, magnesium, malic acid, 5-HTP, and increased fluids.

I asked Marissa to eat three regular meals and three nutritious snacks each day. Instead of a diet, we discussed various food groups and the benefits of each. She felt comfortable choosing an appropriate amount of carbohydrate, fat, and protein for her caloric needs, and we agreed to reassess her progress in two weeks. I also showed her the bottles containing the supplements and reviewed with her the substances they contained. Although Marissa stated she was not a very good pill taker," she agreed to take them consistently as recommended for the next several weeks.

The MultiMax formula from Health*Max* is the specialty multiple vitamin supplement I recommended to Marissa. It contains high-quality ingredients designed for optimal absorption and bioavailability. MultiMax is very well tolerated by my patients, contrary to the many over-the-counter brands that can make people feel nauseated after they ingest them.

I prescribe six to eight MultiMax tablets per day for my patients. I also highly recommend that they read the Supplement Facts on the label (the listing is required by law). This notice specifies the number of tablets per serving and the amount of each nutrient supplied in a *complete serving* (not an individual pill). One serving size of MultiMax consists of eight tablets. A complete serving of MultiMax contains the nutrients listed below. Supplements are measured either in milligrams (mg), micrograms (mcg), or International Units (IU).

TABLE 6.1

Supplement Facts

I.	Vitamin A*	
	25% as retinyl acetate	5,000 IU
	75% as beta-carotene	15,000 IU
II.	Vitamin D (cholecalciferol)	400 IU
III.	Vitamin E (D-alpha tocopheryl succinate)	100 IU
IV.	Vitamin C (ascorbic acid)	1,200 mg
V.	Thiamine (vitamin B_1)(mononitrate)	30 mg
VI.	Riboflavin (vitamin B_2)	34 mg
VII.	Niacin (vitamin B_3)	420 mg
VIII.	Pantothenic Acid (vitamin B_5)	200 mg
IX.	Pyridoxine HCl (vitamin B_6)	40mg
X.	Folic acid	800 mcg
XI.	Cyanocobalamin (vitamin B_{12})	200 mcg
XII.	Biotin	200 mcg
XIII.	Betaine HC	175 mg
XIV.	Choline (bitartate)	125 mg
XV.	Inositol	120 mg
XVI.	PABA (para-aminobenzoic acid)	50 mg
XVII.	Citrus bioflavanoid complex	100 mg
XVIII.	Calcium (citrate, glycinate,	
	microcrystalline hydroxyapatite)	500 mg
XIX.	Magnesium (glycinate, citrate)	250 mg
XX.	Potassium (aspartate)	99 mg
XXI.	Iodine (potassium iodide)	150 mcg
XXII.	Chromium (dinicotinate glycinate)	200 mcg
XXIII.	Selenium (aspartate)	200 mcg
XXIV.	Molybdenum (aspartate)	100 mcg
XXV.	Vanadium (vanadium sulfate)	39 mg
XXVI.	L-glutamine	100 mg
XXVII.	Quercetin (dihydrate)	25 mg
XXVIII.	Alpha-carotene	132 mcg
XXIX.	Cryptoxanthin	32 mcg
XXX.	Zeaxanthin	26 mcg
XXXI.	Lutein	20 mcg
XXXII.	SOD precursor blend	
	Copper (lysinate)	2 mg
	Zinc (glycinate, histidinate)	20 mg
	Manganese (glycinate)	1 mg

(*Pregnant women should not exceed 5,000 IU total intake of vitamin A each day due to increased toxicity and potential birth defects.)

Marissa looked at the size of the pills and wrinkled her nose. "These are huge!" At her follow-up visit one month later, however, Marissa said that she had difficulty swallowing the pills only for the first two days. Once she had gotten used to them, she added one tablet each day, as I had asked, until she reached a total of eight spread throughout the day.

In just the four weeks since her first visit, Marissa had begun to feel much better. She had much more energy (due to the DHEA and the multiple vitamin supplement), less muscle pain and spasm (from the effects of magnesium and malic acid), and she was sleeping better (due to 5-HTP) and had much more coping ability. She felt generally happier than she had on her initial visit—and she had lost six pounds over the four-week interim!

Marissa's improvement continued over the next eight months. She also had some pleasant, unexpected surprises. She noticed that she had not come down with any acute illnesses since beginning to take the vitamin and mineral supplement. Normally, she would have been sick four or five times during an eight-month period. Marissa also could not believe the increase in her energy, stamina, and sense of well-being. "I really didn't realize how important vitamins and minerals are," she told me. "I have noticed so many differences in how I feel."

Pills vs. Meals

Today it can be tricky to get the full complement of vitamins, minerals, micronutrients, and other substances that are the foundation of good nutrition. Few women perform the degree of physical labor that would offset the high calorie intake required to obtain all the nutrients required every day. Some people survive on a steady diet of fast food, which is notoriously long on fat and calories and short on nutrient-rich fresh fruits and vegetables. Others live an especially nutritionally demanding, high-stress life. For these people a multiple vitamin, consumed in conjunction with a reasonable diet, can bridge the gap.

Beyond that, supplementation can become tricky—especially for women who choose to take large amounts of one vitamin or mineral. For instance:

- The right amount of vitamin A fosters good vision, but too much can destroy the liver and be harmful to a fetus.
- Too much niacin can cause flushing; too little can lead to the gum disease called pellagra.

- Too much choline can cause gastrointestinal distress and fishy body odor. Too little may result in memory problems.
- Taken at conception and in the early weeks of pregnancy, folic acid can help prevent spina bifida, a serious, potentially fatal birth defect. It also helps to disarm homocysteine, the catalyst for early heart disease and atherosclerosis. But if you take too much folic acid at once, it can interfere with the absorption of zinc.

It is tempting to think that one food, vitamin, or supplement can provide complete health and wellness. But it is not that simple. It is really the synergy between all of the vitamins, minerals, and micronutrients that makes it possible for the body to function at its best.

The fact is, vitamins and minerals alone do not provide body energy. Food supplies energy. Vitamins and minerals facilitate the release of that energy by helping the body to digest, absorb, and metabolize nutrients. That means vitamins and mineral supplements by themselves do not provide adequate nutrition and cannot substitute for it.

The Essential Vitamins

Nutritionists recognize 13 essential vitamins. These fall into two categories: water soluble and fat soluble.

The water-soluble vitamins (vitamin C and the eight B vitamins) are absorbed directly into the bloodstream. Since they cannot be stored, the kidneys excrete any excess. This safety mechanism protects the body from accumulating a toxic supply of these substances. It also means that our supply of these vitamins must be replenished daily.

The fat-soluble vitamins (A, D, E, and K) are found in the oily or fatty portions of food and can be absorbed only in the presence of dietary fat. For instance, vegetable oils are the main source of vitamin E in the American diet. They enter the bloodstream via the intestinal wall and can lodge in fat-storage sites in the body. So if you take more of these vitamins than your body needs, they will be stored. And if you take high levels of these vitamins in the form of supplements, they could have toxic effects.

RDAs, RDIs, and DRVs

The commonly used term RDA stands for Recommended Dietary Allowance. Recommended dietary allowances of nutrients can be very confusing to many patients. The Food and Nutrition Board (which reports to the National Research Council of the National Academy of Sciences) establishes the RDAs. RDAs are *not* established to suggest the *optimal* intake for an individual, but rather to serve as community standards and guidelines for overall nutrition adequate to *prevent deficiency diseases*. Looking at the label on a bottle of vitamins will reveal that it now lists a "% Daily Value" or "% DV" next to a given ingredient if a daily value has been established. Many clinicians and research scientists recommend vitamins in a therapeutic dose that can be much higher than the RDA.

Another value you may encounter is the RDI, which is the Reference Daily Intake for vitamins and minerals. The RDI was established in 1990 by the National Food Labeling Education Act (NFLEA). The RDI refers to the level of a nutrient that meets the needs of practically all healthy people as calculated by a weighed average of age, gender, pregnancy, and lactation.

The Daily Reference Value, or DRV, is another guideline for consumer use. Food labels now list standard suggested intakes of fat (total and saturated), cholesterol, sodium, total carbohydrate, and dietary fiber for diets consisting of 2,000 and 2,500 total calories per day (the DRV). Labels for individual foods are also required to state the "% daily value" for each of these components (based on a 2,000-calorie diet) contained in a single serving. Such labeling makes it much easier to know what you are eating and to compare the nutritional values of different food choices. It also helps you keep track of just what is in the food you are eating. (An excellent resource for detailed discussion of RDAs, RDIs, and DRVs is found in the book *Clinical Nutrition: A Functional Approach* published by the Institute for Functional Medicine, Inc.)

Like the RDAs, RDIs and DRVs are based on the minimum values needed to prevent severe deficiency diseases. These values usually fall short of what is recommended by leaders in the field of nutritional medicine to optimize health. As each of us has different and individualized needs with regard to nutrition, we must use therapeutic nutrition—including supplements—wisely, and in doses that are beneficial for our unique needs.

Antioxidants

Beyond releasing and helping with metabolizing the energy in food, some vitamins—specifically, vitamin C, vitamin E, lipoic acid, CoQ10, glutathione, beta-carotene, and carotenoids, as well as the minerals selenium, copper, and manganese—do double duty as antioxidants. These substances are believed to play a role in preventing heart disease and cancer as well as arthritis, atherosclerosis, and impaired immune systems. They appear to facilitate the cleanup of oxygen-free radicals that are released as cells burn the oxygen they need to metabolize carbohydrates, fats, and proteins.

While all of the substances I mentioned are technically antioxidants, they are not interchangeable. For instance, vitamin E appears to offer protection against heart disease, while carotenoids appear to shield the retina from degeneration. As with other vitamins, women who eat a balanced diet rich in foods containing a wide variety of antioxidants appear to gain the greatest benefits from these substances. Later in this chapter I will list the foods that contain large amounts of various antioxidants.

Beyond Antioxidants

Food also contains phytochemicals, substances manufactured by plants as protection against damage from free radicals, viruses, extremes of heat and cold, and rough handling. Phytochemicals appear to transfer some of their protective ability to the cells of people who eat them.

While phytochemicals are classified as nonnutrient constituents of food—they have no calories and are not needed for normal function—they do appear to play a role in good health. For instance, they boost the activity of enzymes that act as blocking agents to prevent toxins from reaching or reacting with vulnerable tissues. Some phytochemicals help protect against heart disease by hunting down free radicals and preventing formation of artery-clogging clots; others attack and remove substances that cause cancer.

Darker and more colorful fruits and vegetables are the best source for these beneficial natural compounds.

Vitamins and Minerals: The Basics

The following information is designed to give you specific information on individual vitamins and minerals. I will describe the body systems primarily affected, tell you the recommended dosage for supplementation, and list the foods that contain the greatest quantities of each nutrient.

Remember that many vitamins and minerals work together, so loading up on one (especially the fat-soluble ones) to the exclusion of others can have unintended results. At the same time, loading up on excessive water-soluble vitamins is a waste, as the extra intake beyond what is needed by the body will just excreted in the urine.

The suggestions for supplemental intake are general recommendations only. Specific needs or conditions may exist in individuals that would require significantly more of a particular nutritional supplement or supplements. Use the following discussion as a guideline and modify it based on consultation with a health care provider.

Vitamin A

For women vitamin A is especially important in keeping the skin moist and elastic and helping maintain cell structure and integrity, especially in the eyes and vagina. It also helps hair, skin, and gums stay healthy. It is a key component in the process of detoxification, helping to rid the body of toxic chemicals and by-products of metabolism.

Vitamin A is essential in the manufacture of medications containing retinoids. Retinoids (like the popular retin-A) have been proven beneficial when applied to the skin to treat acne, sun damage, skin diseases such as psoriasis, and wounds.

Vitamin A is found in liver, whole and fortified milk, and eggs. Carotenoids that can be used to make a type of vitamin A are abundant in orange fruits and vegetables and in green leafy vegetables.

Cautions: Excess vitamin A intake may be toxic and may increase the risk of birth defects. Pregnant women and women who may become pregnant should not exceed 5,000 IU of preformed vitamin A (retinyl acetate or retinyl palmitate) per day. It is also recommended that children under four should not regularly consume more than 2,500 IU per day.

Women who are taking oral contraceptives, who smoke, or who are taking estrogen may need higher levels of vitamin A. Because large doses of vitamin E may inhibit the action of vitamin A, women who take vitamin E may need additional vitamin A.

Recommended daily intake for vitamin A (retinyl acetate): 5,000 IU

Beta-carotene

Beta-carotene (also called provitamin A because it is converted into a form of vitamin A) may help prevent a variety of health issues facing women, including breast and lung cancer. Beta-carotene is also believed to reduce premenstrual mastodynia (breast soreness) and prevent cell aging and atherosclerosis as a result of its antioxidant properties. As an antioxidant, beta-carotene prevents damage to tissues by free radicals. Many supplements use beta-carotene as a source for vitamin A because the body will convert it to vitamin A—but only if there is a need for it.

Beta-carotene is found in dark green, dark yellow, and orange vegetables such as spinach, collard greens, broccoli, carrots, peppers, and sweet potatoes, as well as in yellow fruits such as apricots and peaches.

Recommended daily intake for beta-carotene: 15,000 IU

The B Vitamins

You should always take B vitamin supplements as a complex. Since they work in combination, a complex ensures that you will ingest the appropriate balance for gaining the maximum benefit.

B_1/THIAMINE Every woman knows how important collagen is for youthful skin. B_1 fosters collagen-rich connective tissues as well as helping to keep mucus membranes healthy while maintaining smooth muscle. It also may reduce fatigue and improve mood and reaction time, and has been known as the energy vitamin because it acts to speed the chemical reactions that are required to process carbohydrates. Thiamine is commonly used for dementia, confusion, nerve damage, alcoholism, chronic pain, and stress.

Vitamin B_1 is found in wheat germ, peanuts, sunflower seeds, pine nuts, soybeans, split peas, beans, seafood, whole grains, and unmilled rice.

Cautions: Enzymes in raw fish, coffee, and tea damage thiamine. B_1 absorption is decreased when a folic acid deficiency is present.

Recommended daily intake for B_1/thiamine: 2–10 mg

B₂ / RIBOFLAVIN Vitamin B_2 is important for a woman's overall growth as well as for red blood cell formation and antibody production. Riboflavin is also necessary for healthy hair, nails, and mucous membranes. It is an important B vitamin involved in the body's defense system against oxidative damage. Riboflavin is responsible for the characteristic smell, taste, and yellow color of the B vitamins. An inadequate supply of riboflavin can lead to fatigue, muscle weakness, and decreased energy.

Riboflavin is found in meat, eggs, legumes, fruits, poultry, green leafy vegetables, and fish.

Cautions: Women with low thyroid levels or who exercise excessively or drink alcohol may need additional B_2.

Recommended daily intake for B₂/riboflavin: 20–50 mg

B₃ / NIACIN Vitamin B_3, or niacin, is an important element in the production of most of women's sex hormones. Niacin also helps with overall circulation and lowers bad (LDL) cholesterol while raising the good (HDL) cholesterol. Studies have found that 1 gram of B_3 each day decreases the risk of recurrent heart attacks. This is an especially important issue for postmenopausal women. Niacin also plays an important role in the activity of insulin helping to prevent diabetes. Too little niacin is associated with dermatitis, dementia, diarrhea, arthritis, memory problems, and depression.

Niacin is found in meat, fish, poultry, brewer's yeast, rice bran, wheat bran, and peanuts. Because B_3 is largely unavailable in a vegetarian diet, non-meat eaters should consider supplements.

Cautions: Women with ulcers, liver disease, gout, or heart disease should talk with their doctors before taking B_3 supplements. Too much niacin can cause dilation of the arteries, which can lead to fainting or sweating. It can also impair liver function, which is why periodic liver function tests are recommended.

Recommended daily intake for B₃/niacin: 20–50 mg

B₅ / PANTOTHENIC ACID Vitamin B_5 is known as an antistress vitamin. Pantothenic acid is important for maintaining a woman's adrenal gland hormones and may have an overall affect on energy. Pantothenic acid is involved in making several amino acids—the precursors to important proteins in the body. A low level of vitamin B_5 can cause gastrointestinal problems like colitis, fatigue, increased infections, allergies, and problems with detoxification.

Vitamin B_5 is found in whole wheat, beans, freshwater fish, meats, milk, and fresh vegetables.

Cautions: B_5 may cause diarrhea and water retention at high levels of supplementation.

Recommended daily intake for B_5/pantothenic acid: 200 mg

B_6 / PYRIDOXINE Vitamin B_6 consists of three compounds: pyridoxine, pyridoxamine, and pyridoxal. This vitamin is involved in at least 100 different body reactions and in the production of key proteins. Along with folate and B_{12}, B_6 may be helpful in decreasing homocysteine, an amino acid associated with aggressive heart disease and hardening of the arteries. B_6 is frequently depleted by excessive alcohol consumption.

Vitamin B_6 is found in chicken, fish, kidney, liver, pork, eggs, brown rice, soybeans, oats, whole-wheat products, peanuts, and walnuts. It is also found in carrots, spinach, and wheat germ.

Cautions: Excessive doses can lead to toxicity. Do not use vitamin B_6 with levodopa. B_6 may decrease blood levels of certain antiseizure medications.

Recommended daily intake for B_6/pyridoxine: 5–50 mg

VITAMIN B_{12} / CYANOCOBALAMIN Vitamin B_{12} is necessary for the manufacture of red blood cells. Therefore, this vitamin is essential for the prevention of anemia, a concern for every premenopausal woman. B_{12} is also important for the overall function of the nervous system and for the metabolism of folic acid, another B vitamin essential to preventing the birth defect spina bifida. As we discussed in the section on vitamin B_6, the combination of B_6, B_{12}, and folic acid may also help to decrease homocysteine, an amino acid associated with heart disease, the primary cause of death in women. Alcohol and gout medications may interfere with B_{12} absorption.

B_{12} is found mainly in animal products, especially liver and other organ meats. It is also found in clams, oysters, diary products, seafood, eggs, tofu, and seaweed.

Cautions: B_{12} deficiencies are common in strict vegetarians and people with age-related loss of stomach acid or pernicious anemia.

Recommended daily intake for B_{12}/cyanocobalamin: 200 mcg

Biotin

Biotin is necessary for the metabolism of carbohydrates, proteins, and fats. Biotin is needed for healthy nails and hair. Biotin is also beneficial in glucose regulation by making insulin more sensitive, potentially avoiding diabetes. Biotin is found in saltwater fish, cooked egg yolks, soybeans, poultry, whole grains, and yeast. Seizures, poor muscle tone and weakness, unsteady gait, alopecia (hair loss), dermatitis, depression, and hallucinations are associated with a low level of biotin.

Cautions: Biotin absorption is inhibited by sulfa drugs, antibiotics, and raw egg whites.

Recommended daily intake for biotin: 200 mcg

Para-aminobenzoic Acid (PABA)

PABA, which helps to metabolize proteins, is thought to help prevent abnormal fibrous tissue from being formed in the body. PABA is also important in the production of red blood cells. When applied to the skin PABA acts as a sunscreen, although allergic reactions are common when it is used in this way.

PABA is found in molasses, whole grains, and organ meats such as liver and kidney.

Cautions: Absorption of PABA may be inhibited by sulfa drugs, estrogen, and alcohol.

Recommended daily intake for PABA: 50 mg

Inositol

Inositol removes fat from the arteries and liver, making it essential for a woman's long-term good health by aiding in the prevention of heart disease. Inositol hexaniacinate has been shown to work like niacin but without all the side effects (fainting, sweating, impaired liver function). Inositol is necessary for healthy brain function, and it also contributes to healthy hair.

Inositol is found in fruit, milk, whole grains, and meat. Estrogen, caffeine, and alcohol inhibit inositol absorption.

Recommended daily intake for inositol: 120 mg

Choline

Choline plays a crucial role in nervous system and brain functioning, including memory. It is also important for gallbladder and liver function and performs a critical function in fat metabolism.

Choline is found in egg yolks, soybeans, meat, milk, and whole grains.

Cautions: Excess consumption of choline may result in a gastrointestinal distress and fishy body odor.

Recommended daily intake for choline: 125 mg

Folic Acid/Folate

Folic acid is essential to the production of red blood cells and hormones, as well as to DNA synthesis. As previously mentioned, folic acid, along with vitamins B_6 and B_{12}, may help decrease homocysteine, an amino acid associated with heart disease. When taken during early pregnancy, folic acid also helps prevent the potentially deadly birth defect spina bifida.

For women taking birth control pills, folic acid supplements may improve the occurrence of dysplasia or abnormal cell growth detected by a Pap smear. For older women with memory or emotional disorders, early research may indicate that folic acid yields some improvement.

Folic acid is found in yeast, liver and other organ meats, green and leafy vegetables, some fruit, and in fortified foods containing added folic acid. But be aware that cooking destroys up to 95% of folic acid and alcohol interferes with its absorption.

Cautions: Women who are pregnant or thinking of becoming pregnant should talk with their doctors about folic acid supplements. People taking anticonvulsant drugs should talk with their doctors about the effect folic acid may have on absorption. High levels of folic acid may interfere with the absorption of zinc.

Recommended daily intake for folic acid: 400–800 mcg

Vitamin C

Vitamin C helps metabolize amino acids to form epinephrine, a substance released during periods of stress. Vitamin C is required for the formation of collagen, the fibrous structural protein that supports teeth, bones, skin, and cell walls. It also acts as an extracellular antioxidant to protect cells from diseases such as cancers of the lung, stomach, and esophagus. It also promotes the absorption of iron and may reduce the severity of colds. Low levels are associated with recurrent infections, colds, poor wound healing, and fatigue.

Vitamin C is found in citrus fruits and strawberries, broccoli, cabbage, peppers, tomatoes, and fortified breakfast cereals.

Cautions: Vitamin C can be important for women who are taking birth control pills or who are on estrogen; are pregnant or breast-feeding; or who smoke, drink alcohol, or have undergone surgery. Vitamin C can be depleted by antibiotics, corticosteroids, and ibuprofen. At high doses vitamin C has been linked to kidney stones and gout. Large amounts of chewable vitamin C can damage tooth enamel.

Recommended daily intake for vitamin C: 500–2,000 mg

Vitamin D

In combination with calcium and phosphorus, vitamin D promotes women's ability to grow strong bones, prevents bone softening and osteoporosis, and may lower blood pressure. Vitamin D tells the kidneys not to release calcium and phosphate into the urine, allowing more of these compounds to be available to make bone. Nerves, muscles, and blood are all dependent on adequate levels of vitamin D.

Vitamin D is made out of cholesterol in our skin when it is exposed to sunlight. Vitamin D is found in fish liver oils, fatty fish, egg yolks, and fortified milk.

Cautions: Sunscreens and sun-damaged or darkly pigmented skin retard vitamin D synthesis. Vitamin D can be blocked by anticonvulsant treatments as well as some liver and kidney diseases.

Recommended daily intake for vitamin D: 400 IU

Vitamin E

Women who get adequate vitamin E may find that it relieves hot flashes, breast soreness related to menopause, fibrocystic breast disease, the occurrence of breast tumors, and the symptoms of PMS. As one of the most important antioxidants, vitamin E helps protect cells against some diseases, including cancer. It also may slow the progress of Alzheimer's disease. Low levels of vitamin E can lead to difficulty digesting and absorbing fatty foods.

Vitamin E is found in soybeans; corn, cottonseed, and safflower oils;

and products made from these oils (for example, margarine and shortening), wheat germ, brown rice, sesame seeds, nuts, and green leafy vegetables. It is also found in liver, haddock, mackerel, and herring.

Recommended daily intake for vitamin E: 100–800 IU

Vitamin K

Vitamin K aids in building bones and preventing osteoporosis by synthesizing proteins found in bones. It also synthesizes at least six proteins required for blood clotting.

Vitamin K is found in broccoli, brussels sprouts, watercress, parsley, collard and mustard greens, and kale. It is also contained in tofu made with calcium carbonate, sardines and salmon with bones, fortified orange juice, green tea, butter, liver, bacon, and coffee.

Cautions: Talk with your doctor about vitamin K if you are taking a blood thinner such as Coumadin as it can counteract the effects of type of medication.

Recommended daily intake for vitamin K: 150–500 mcg

Coenzyme Q10 (CoQ10)

Every cell in a woman's body uses CoQ10 to produce chemical energy. In particular, the heart needs CoQ10, and its use has been linked to increase efficiency of the heart muscle's performance. Decreased levels of CoQ10 are associated with heart failure. In combination with vitamin E, CoQ10 works as a potent antioxidant that helps protect women from atherosclerosis. There may be a link between CoQ10 deficiency and breast cancer. One study has connected CoQ10 to improved physical performance and recovery after exertion.

CoQ10 is found in organ meats, sardines, mackerel, beef, peanuts, and soy oil.

Cautions: Some drugs used for lowering cholesterol interfere with CoQ10 absorption, so if you are taking such medications you should talk with your doctor about taking a supplement.

Recommended daily intake for CoQ10: 50–150 mg

Boron

The role of boron in influencing the metabolism of calcium, magnesium, vitamin D, and phosphorus is still under study. It is a trace mineral women need to build strong bones and healthy joints.

Boron is found in grapes, raisins, apples, nuts, cider, and beer. It is also found in green leafy vegetables and grains.

Recommended daily intake for boron: 3–9 mg

Calcium

For all women, calcium is the foundation for building and maintaining strong bones. Calcium also plays a role in maintaining good blood pressure, and it may protect the colon from increased cell proliferation caused by fat and bile acids.

Women who meet their RDA for both calcium and magnesium reduce their risk of hypertension by 35% compared to those who don't. Calcium also is essential for the muscles to be able to relax and contract.

Calcium is found in dairy and soybean products, green leafy vegetables, canned salmon with bones, mackerel, sardines, raisins, and seaweed. A balance of vitamin D, calcium, and phosphorus is essential for the calcium in dairy products to be absorbed. Alcohol, protein, and foods such as beet greens, spinach, rhubarb, chard, and almonds, which contain oxalic acid, impair calcium absorption.

Cautions: Low levels of estrogen, such as those that occur during perimenopause and menopause, increase calcium loss.

Some medications, including anticoagulants, antiseizure drugs, and long-term use of cortisone, may impede calcium absorption. If you are prone to kidney stones, kidney disease, or heart disease, you should talk with your doctor before taking calcium supplements.

Recommended daily intake for calcium: 500–1,500 mg

Chromium

Chromium helps insulin metabolize fat, turn protein into muscle, and convert sugar into energy. Chromium-activated insulin increases the amount of blood sugar available for energy production nearly twentyfold. ChromeMate is a unique, patented form of biologically active niacin-bound chromium called chromium nicotinate or polynicotinate that dramatically increases the effectiveness of chromium. Researcher has shown that ChromeMate is the safest and most potent form of chromium available as a dietary supplement.

Chromium is found in whole-grain products, processed meats, and bran cereals, brewer's yeast, calf's liver, American cheese, and wheat germ. You can protect the chromium levels in your food by using only stainless steel cookware.

Recommended daily intake for chromium: 400–1,000 mcg

Copper

By oxidizing iron and preventing free-radical formation, copper plays a significant role in heart disease prevention for women. It is a cofactor in many enzyme reactions in the body and is the third most abundant essential trace mineral. Copper helps produce energy and is important in giving the skin its elasticity.

Copper is found in kidneys, soybeans, wheat germ, shellfish, legumes, liver, nuts, and bran.

Cautions: Copper deficiencies are common among people who receive intravenous feeding.

Recommended daily intake for copper: 1.5–3 mg

Iodine

Iodine is important to a woman's overall stamina and well-being. It is one of the minerals that regulates the rate at which energy is released from nutrients. It also is one of two essential thyroid hormones regulating growth, reproduction, nerve and muscle function, synthesis of blood cells, and body temperature. Iodine may also have a role to play in the treatment of fibrocystic breast disease.

Iodine is found in mushrooms, soybeans, summer squash, and garlic. While people who live near the ocean can get iodine from seafood, water, and even ocean mist, the most reliable source is iodized table salt. Brussels sprouts, cabbage, pears, spinach, and turnips may interfere with iodine absorption when eaten in large quantities.

Cautions: When taken in large doses, iodine may cause enlargement of the thyroid gland.

Recommended daily intake for iodine: 150 mcg

Iron

Iron is an essential element in a woman's metabolism. It is used to form the proteins hemoglobin and myoglobin, which carry oxygen to the tissues of the body and muscle. Iron is also involved in making amino acids, hormones, and neurotransmitters and is a key factor in energy production.

Iron is found in meat, fish, and poultry as well as in fortified foods, fruits, vegetables, and juices. Alcohol and vitamin C enhance iron absorption. However, milk, unprocessed grains, coffee, tea, and nuts interfere with iron absorption, and you should avoid taking your supplements with these foods.

Cautions: High levels of iron may increase the risk of heart disease. Both high and low levels may increase the risk of infection. Women who have a tendency to store excess iron should talk with their physicians before taking iron supplements. We recommend ferrous sulfate or iron chelate supplements, which are easy for the body to absorb.

Recommended daily intake for iron: 15 mg

Magnesium

Magnesium works in concert with hundreds of chemical reactions in the body that metabolize food and transmit messages between cells. It is crucial to the function of a woman's bones, heart, muscles, and nerves. Magnesium also helps in the management of hypertension during pregnancy, in treating cardiac arrhythmias, and in managing diabetes. In my practice I recommend it for muscle spasm, headache, abnormal heart rhythms, and constipation.

Magnesium is widely available in unprocessed foods such as nuts, legumes, whole grains, green vegetables, and bananas. High levels of calcium can interfere with magnesium absorption.

Cautions: Large doses of magnesium may be toxic for people with kidney disease. Magnesium absorption also is inhibited by the use of diuretics, so women who take diuretics for congestive heart failure and high blood pressure, alcoholics, some diabetics, and individuals with certain gastrointestinal disorders should talk with their physicians about magnesium supplements.

Recommended daily intake for magnesium: 250 mg

Manganese

Manganese is important for bone formation, growth, and development. Manganese also is important for every woman's energy and protein metabolism. Low levels can be associated with hair loss, skin rashes, fatigue, and decreased nail and hair growth.

Manganese is found in whole-grain and cereal products, eggs, dairy products, nuts, and leafy vegetables.

Cautions: Women who have low manganese levels may be at risk for iron loss due to menstrual bleeding. Absorption of manganese is inhibited by large amounts of calcium, phosphorus, magnesium, phytates from whole grains, tannins, and oxalic acid.

Recommended daily intake for manganese: 2–5 mg

Molybdenum

A component of several enzymes, molybdenum facilitates fat metabolism and is required for iron utilization and detoxification.

Molybdenum is found in dairy products, dried legumes, organ meats, cereals, and baked goods.

Cautions: Excessive molybdenum can interfere with calcium absorption.

Recommended daily intake for molybdenum: 75–250 mcg

Phosphorus

Phosphorus is integral to the formation of every cell in a woman's body—especially bone cells. Phosphorus also plays a role in growth, energy metabolism, maintaining the balance between the acid and base status in bodily fluid, lipid transport, and the traffic of nutrients in and out of cells.

Half the phosphorus in the American diet comes from milk, meat, poultry, and fish. Phosphorus is also found in cereals and convenience foods.

Cautions: Phosphorus is readily available, so most Americans easily exceed the RDA. This can be problematic for women concerned about osteoporosis, since high levels of phosphorus are associated with excess calcium excretion and bone loss. Excess phosphorus may suppress the synthesis of vitamin D, another key player in bone formation. Antacids containing aluminum hydroxide may inhibit phosphorus absorption, so make certain to read the label before consuming.

Recommended daily intake for phosphorus: 800 mg

Potassium

While potassium is best known for its ability to reduce the risk of strokes and maintain good blood pressure, it is also necessary for the transmission of nerve impulses and muscle contraction. A potassium deficiency can cause weakness and listlessness, and may trigger extra heartbeats that can prevent the heart from pumping normally.

Potassium is found in many unprocessed foods such as fruits, vegetables, legumes, and fresh meats. Alcohol and coffee promote the loss of potassium from the body.

Cautions: Women with diabetes or kidney disease should avoid potassium supplements because their bodies may not be able to excrete large amounts.

Recommended daily intake for potassium: 2,000 mg

Selenium

As a component of an enzyme with antioxidant properties, selenium promotes a woman's heart health. It also may free up vitamin E for other tasks and reduce the risk of cancer.

Selenium is found in meats (especially seafood, kidney, and liver) as well as in egg yolks, mushrooms, garlic, cereals, and grains.

Recommended daily intake for selenium: 50–200 mcg

Sodium

Sodium regulates the volume of fluid in a woman's body, maintains the body's acid-base balance, transmits nerve signals, and helps muscles contract.

Sodium is found in table salt, processed food, baked goods, meat, and dairy products. People in general eat far more salt than they should, which is part of the reason diseases like high blood pressure are on the rise in virtually every corner of the world. The National High Blood Pressure Education Program recommends a daily consumption of no more than 2,400 mg of sodium, about 6 grams of table salt. I recommend consuming far less—

500 mg—since salt contributes to a variety of problems related to stress, including high blood pressure, heart disease, stroke, and water weight.

Cautions: People who have been diagnosed with high blood pressure should follow their physician's recommendations regarding sodium intake.

Recommended daily intake for sodium: 500 mg

Zinc

A vital component of the enzymes involved in more than 100 metabolic processes, zinc is crucial to women's growth and development, immune function, blood clotting, wound healing, and the production of the active form of vitamin A in visual pigments.

Zinc is found in meat, liver, eggs, and seafood (especially oysters). The zinc in whole grains is a less available form than that found in meat. Both breast milk and zinfandel wine enhance the availability of zinc.

Cautions: Older women are particularly at risk for marginal zinc deficiency. This is because they consume less than two-thirds of the RDA for zinc, and their bodies do not absorb zinc well. In addition, they are more likely to develop conditions that interfere with the absorption and metabolism of zinc (for example, diabetes and gastrointestinal disorders) and to take medications (such as diuretics) that increase zinc excretion. Supplemental fiber, calcium, and iron also may block zinc absorption.

Recommended daily intake for zinc: 20–30 mg

Shopping for Supplements

Americans spend billions of dollars each year on dietary supplements. A 1999 Gallup study found that one of every two adults use nutritional supplements. These range from your basic daily multivitamin to exotic concoctions guaranteed to do everything from improve your sex life to help you sleep at night.

Once the exclusive purview of the local health food store, even the major drugstore chains have gotten into the action, marketing supplements under their own names. You can now buy supplements on the Internet or through a myriad of other distribution channels.

Know What You're Buying

Research is essential in buying supplements. Here are some of the most important things to keep in mind:

- Shop around, and look for good value. The most expensive may not necessarily be the best.
- Know what you are buying, and avoid getting sidetracked by similar-sounding products. For instance, one supplement may include a label listing of 100 mg zinc picolinate, while another lists 100 mg zinc (picolinate). In the first instance, the measure reflects the combined volume of the two substances; in the second it reflects only the amount of zinc, so the first product contains less zinc than the second.
- Be aware that your body may not be utilizing the full strength of the supplements you are taking. In the mid-1980s a study at the University of Maryland found that many calcium supplements didn't break down when placed in a stomach-acid-like substance. To address this issue, the National Osteoporosis Foundation recommends testing calcium supplements to be sure they break down sufficiently. Just place the tablet in six ounces of vinegar for 30 minutes, stirring occasionally. If the tablet doesn't completely disintegrate, it probably will not break down in your stomach.
- Keep an eye out for so-called other ingredients. These range from food coloring and preservatives to fillers. Sometimes these substances can cause reactions you weren't expecting. For instance, people who are allergic to milk may have a reaction to a supplement that contains dry milk as the suspension or as a filler. Extra ingredients, like sugar and starch, may not always be bad, however. Although no one wants to consume unneeded ingredients, some added elements may help tablets disintegrate more quickly. That can make them more easily utilized by the body. And a small amount of sugar in a chewable supplement can make it more palatable.
- Beware of marketing gimmicks. Customers looking to reduce their cancer risk may be drawn to expensive products that tout supplements and vitamins containing antioxidants. But before you buy, compare the dosages of these specialty packages with

the antioxidants in your multiple vitamin. You may find that the contents are the same, but your multiple vitamin may be cheaper.

- Natural is not always better. On a cellular level, your body can't distinguish between a manufactured supplement and one that is a plant extract. An exception is vitamin E, for which the natural form is more chemically active than the synthetic form. I always recommend natural vitamin E to my patients.
- Promoting alleged innovation is the oldest advertising gimmick in the world. But new isn't necessarily better or even useful.
- Check the date and safety seal. Just like milk and mayonnaise, supplements can spoil or lose their effectiveness, so always check the expiration date. Make sure your containers are sealed shut when you buy them.
- Just like medications, vitamin and mineral supplements should be stored in a cool dry place. Many deteriorate when exposed to light or heat.

CHAPTER SEVEN

Step 3: Taming the Tiger

If you scored low in the Taming the Tiger section of The Stress Cure Inventory, you are definitely not alone.

Most of my patients understand the importance of stress management. They even know about many of the traditional stress management techniques before I have a chance to describe them. The problem is that too many women simply do not give themselves permission to put these techniques into practice. They just aren't used to taking care of themselves or putting their own needs before the needs of others.

I am here to tell you that if you want to maximize your health and well-being, this kind of thinking must change.

In this chapter I'll explain how to begin to make the behavioral changes that will help you manage the stress in your life. We'll start with some stress reduction techniques that take only a little time and effort. I will give you some suggestions for reducing stress by enhancing the energy of your mind, body, and spirit. A large part of this chapter is devoted to a detailed discussion of meditation, which in my personal and professional experience is the most effective behavioral method of controlling stress. Meditation, along with the other stress-reducing measures in this book, can help keep episodes of stress from becoming chronic, allowing the body to replenish its reserves of DHEA and properly use the supplements you are taking. I will also describe several other techniques for relieving stress.

Read this chapter with an open mind, and take the time to try out my suggestions. Soon you will become conscious of the ways you have been taunting your "stress tiger." From that point on it won't take long to develop the habits you need to tame the beast!

Energy-Draining Behaviors

Some stressful events in our lives, such as losing a job or becoming ill, are thrown at us without advance notice. We may feel that we have no control over them. Others are a result of the choices we make on a daily basis. For instance, if you decide not to fold the laundry after it is washed, you may feel stressed when you cannot find a pair of matching socks in the pile. We do have power over those types of stressors.

Believe it or not, it is possible for you to live your life in ways that give you power over even those stressors that you may feel are out of your control. For instance, if you lose your job, if you have maintained a reasonable level of spending, you will probably have enough savings to tide you over until you get a new job. If you have been eating right, exercising, and getting high-quality sleep, your immune system will be better equipped to fight off disease. You may not be able to eliminate the stressor altogether, but you may be able to control the magnitude of its effect.

Below are some behaviors that may be breaking down your mind, body, and spirit and making it difficult for you to manage stress. Within each category, I will also offer suggestions for energy enhancers: things you can do to replenish your reserves and build energy and stamina to resist the effects of stress.

Mind energy drains
- Too much television
- Excessive exposure to the news media (television, radio, newspapers)
- Spending time around demanding people
- Negative self-talk
- Worry
- A cluttered environment
- Financial concerns and overspending
- Unfinished business
- Avoiding conflict

Mind energy enhancers

- Reading and/or listening to inspirational or stimulating books or tapes
- Spending time with friends and family who enhance your life
- Securing a positive financial status and maintaining a reasonable level of spending
- Maintaining an environment that is neat, clean, and well organized
- Seeking conflict resolution
- "Resistive scheduling" (a phrase I use to describe the conscious effort not to fill up every little time slot but to leave buffer room for the unexpected)

Body energy drains

- Smoking
- Alcohol
- Drugs
- Poor diet
- Sugar
- Caffeine
- Food additives
- Lack of exercise
- Sedentary lifestyle
- Being overweight
- Insufficient sleep
- Excessive time around high-energy electrical appliances, especially computers and printers
- Constant rushing
- Environmental toxins, including certain food contaminants

Body energy enhancers

- Nutritious food
- Abundant (good-quality) water
- High-quality vitamin supplements
- Light
- Exercise in all forms (cardiovascular, stretching, weight training)
- Plenty of sleep
- Doing things at your own pace

- Various types of energy work such as yoga
- Therapeutic techniques such as massage
- Relaxing baths
- Hugs

Spirit energy drains

- Not speaking your mind (for fear of hurting someone's feelings, making someone angry, etc.)
- Pushing yourself to do things you do not want to do
- Staying in a job you dislike
- Staying in an unhealthy relationship

Spirit energy enhancers

- Saying only what you believe to be the truth
- Doing everything with love
- Practicing gratitude
- Focusing on what you want instead of don't want
- Focusing on what you have instead of don't have
- Saying no to anything that's not for your highest good
- Listening to and following your inner guidance
- Spending time in nature
- Having fun
- Praying
- Identifying your dream and trying to follow it
- Listening to or creating uplifting music
- Meditating

Meditate to Reduce Stress

There are many methods of stress reduction, but the most effective I have seen is meditation.

Meditation is a form of stress reduction that promotes a deep state of relaxation including slower breathing, slower heart rate, appearance of alpha waves on an EEG (electroencephalogram, which measures brain waves), decreased oxygen consumption, and decreased metabolic rate.

People commonly misperceive meditation as an inward journey for the self-absorbed, an indulgence for those who do not have to work long hours or tend to the needs of others. But the concept of meditation is much simpler than this stereotype, and its benefits are much more practical than many people imagine.

To meditate is to quiet your mind. Meditation allows us to experience silence without thoughts, dilemmas, emotions, to-do lists, obligations, or fears. Research has shown that meditation reduces a woman's heart rate, blood pressure, and adrenaline levels. Meditation also has been shown to improve memory, concentration, and learning.

People who meditate are not necessarily striving to reach a higher state of mind. They are being mindful of the present moment. Individuals who meditate frequently report feelings of inner silence, peacefulness, and effortlessness. When they clear their minds and focus on their breathing, people who meditate find that daily worries and distractions melt away. Afterward they feel focused and in touch with their bodies, and the state of calm they achieve affects the rest of their day.

Julie is one of my patients who meditates successfully. She told me, "I begin every morning, just after I wake up. I sit in a soft chair in our living room—one of the only times I ever get to sit in this peaceful room—and begin my 15- to 20-minute morning meditation. It helps me begin the day with a sense of inner peace and balance."

Mornings weren't always so peaceful for Julie. Prior to meditating, she felt panicked immediately upon awakening. Her heart would pound ferociously, and it occasionally skipped beats. This was due largely, it seems, to the pressures she put on herself.

"I would fly out of bed, start the coffeemaker, yell at the kids to get up, and begin going through the multiple checklists I had in my head for each and every family member," says Julie. "I was the program director. No one had to take responsibility for themselves because I always took responsibility for everyone. Then I would resent everyone for not doing things on his or her own. The time pressure in the morning only made things worse. It took me a long time to see that I was my own worst enemy."

When Julie came to see me about the physical and emotional repercussions of her stressful life, I put her on a stress reduction program built around two meditation sessions per day: 15 minutes in the morning when she awoke, and 15 minutes in the evening before returning from work.

Those two small increments of time have changed Julie's life. Coupled with her daily dose of DHEA, Julie's meditation helps her set the stage for logical, clear thinking.

Julie knows that when she meditates, her mornings are much calmer. She no longer creates morning checklists for her family but gives everyone the opportunity to care for themselves. Meditation helps Julie start her day on her terms, with a sense of control and perspective on what is important.

At the end of her workday Julie closes her office door prior to leaving for the night and sits quietly in a chair. She begins to meditate. Within minutes, she has purged the day's tension from her muscles. Her breathing slows, and she enters a state of mind-body relaxation that allows her to return home with a renewed sense of energy.

The Healing Power of Meditation

Why is meditation such powerful medicine? Meditation initiates a mind-body connection called the relaxation response, which is the opposite of the stress response. Herbert Benson, M.D., a Harvard Medical School researcher, coined the phrase 25 years ago in his book *The Relaxation Response*. Quite simply, relaxation techniques such as meditation trigger a deep state of calm that reduces heart rate, blood pressure, respiratory rate, oxygen consumption, blood flow to skeletal muscles, perspiration, and muscle tension. It is as if you were pushing a reset button on your body or shifting it into a lower gear. Researchers, including Benson, believe that the relaxation response may even trigger self-repair mechanisms in the body.

Benson coauthored a small study that examined what happens in the brain during meditation. Five long-time practitioners of kundalini, an Eastern form of deep meditation, practiced their meditation while being given a brain scan called an MRI. The MRI documented a deep quietude across the entire brain, affecting areas of the brain that control stress-sensitive functions like metabolism and heart rate.

Other studies have shown that when people relax and feel better emotionally (through meditation or other similar techniques), their nervous systems adapt to handle stress better and they become less sensitive to the effects of cortisol. Although people who practice meditation and relaxation techniques have a greater awareness of and reaction to stressful events, it takes less time for them to return to the calmer state they were in before the stressful event took place. In effect, they detect stressors better and dismiss them faster than people who do not meditate.

Contemplation as a Means to Mediation

James Coffin, a personal friend, filmmaker, and Eastern philosophy mentor, has helped me understand the difference between meditation and contemplation. He uses the following example, which I will paraphrase.

We frequently are in a state of desire: We want something; right now we don't have it; we didn't have it yesterday; we need it tomorrow. The thing that we desire can be just about anything: happiness, lack of responsibility, a thin waistline, money, a new car, etc. It is common to live that way: constantly fretting about the past, feeling unsatisfied about the present, and worrying about the future. Restful contemplation (what we commonly call meditation) can help us get to a place (in the strict term, the place is "meditation") that allows the mind to put all of that away, to be closer to the here and now. The Arabic meaning of the word *zero* is "a place where there is nothing." Meditation is your personal zero.

Many of us get wrapped up in the constant turmoil of day-to-day life. Our brains are continually processing a frenzy of information. Eventually, the process can become overwhelming. When we use restful contemplation to reach a state of meditation, we allow the brain to be at rest, to stop vibrating for a while, to stop processing worry, fear, guilt, and the other myriad feelings we continuously experience.

Coffin has also helped me understand that many of us are so focused on goals—buying a new car, buying a house, getting a raise, finding happiness—that we do not enjoy the process of getting there. Many people spend so much energy ruminating about the past and fearing the future that they let the process of life slip by or they spend it in unpleasantness.

Focusing on the Here and Now

As you sit reading this book, understand that right now, at this moment in time, you are all right. You are alive and breathing, probably well fed and clothed. Concentrate on that thought, just for a second. Now for another second. Oh! A third second just passed. Everything is still fine. Do you see what you have just accomplished? You have spent time concentrating on the here and now.

I am hoping that this brief experiment will help you begin to understand how it feels to narrow your focus of experience until you can eventually enjoy living second by second.

How many times have you said, "I have to take a minute to collect my thoughts." Collect them? You have to collect them because there are so many thoughts racing around your mind that you get anxious just trying to think of all the things you are thinking about!

Our society actually promotes and encourages chaotic thinking. Think of the words we use to praise people: "She is such a good multitasker." "He can keep so many balls in the air at once." We truly do create our own levels of stress, and we must be the ones to ultimately recognize it in ourselves and take steps to change our behavior or lifestyle.

In the grand scheme of things the mind seeks happiness. We do ourselves a disservice and actually create more stress for ourselves if we begin vacillating between past concerns and future worries. The constant mental motion of vacillation is taxing. Once you begin to recognize this behavior in yourself and see how quickly those around you use it to escalate their own stresses, it will become easier for you to narrow your focus to the here and now. You will be able to get more enjoyment out of life as you experience the process of getting there rather than merely focusing on the goal.

I feel comfortable talking about this subject because I, too, fall into these stressful patterns of behavior. For that reason I try to practice this type of living as much as possible. It helps to have a mentor, a teacher, a life coach, a friend, or someone who can help you narrow your focus of experience to enjoy each second of life as much as you possible can.

Popular Forms of Meditation

There are two main forms of meditation that have been studied medically: concentrative and awareness.

Concentrative Meditation

Transcendental Meditation (TM) and kundalini are forms of concentrative meditation. This means they focus on a mantra, or a repeated word or word string, that does not have any associated meaning. The mantra is repeated slowly, usually timed with the ebb and flow of deep breathing.

Because the mantra is a collection of syllables that have no direct association, you are less apt to begin connecting thought images with your repetitive sound or phrase. In essence, this allows your brain to quiet down and be at peace. Paradoxically, allowing your mind to quiet down is also a way to reenergize it.

Awareness Meditiation

Awareness, or mindful, meditation is rooted in a Buddhist tradition called *vipassana*. Mindful meditation focuses on becoming aware of thoughts, feelings, and sensations as they arise. It calls for being much more aware of the here and now and really experiencing life at each instant. Mindful meditation was made popular in the U.S. medical arena primarily by Jon Kabat-Zinn, Ph.D., who successfully integrated this technique into his Stress Reduction Clinic at the University of Massachusetts Medical Center.

Which Technique Is Best?

Does one form of meditation work better than another? According to Dr. Herbert Benson, no single technique has a monopoly. Benson's own technique, a nonreligious offshoot of transcendental meditation, involves meditating on a word or phrase that has meaning to the individual. You might choose to meditate on the word *peace,* or *love,* for example. To Benson, transcendental meditation, mindful meditation, yoga, or even reciting the rosary all create the same physiological state of relaxation.

However, according to a 1998 report that examined 597 studies on the effects of mind-body relaxation techniques, TM was found to be far superior to all other forms of meditation and relaxation. Patients practicing TM experienced reduced anxiety and blood pressure, enhanced physiologic relaxation, self-actualization, and psychological outcomes, and decreased use of cigarettes, alcohol, and drugs.

You should not get sidetracked or overwhelmed by wondering which form of meditation is the most effective. In any form, meditation is a very natural activity that can be easily adopted as a routine. Whatever technique feels most comfortable to you is the one you should choose.

Timing Your Session

To benefit fully from any kind of meditation, you should develop a 20-minute routine to be practiced once or twice daily, and a shorter, mini meditation that you can practice anywhere—especially in moments of stress. If I find myself beginning to feel stressed, I simply close my eyes, take in a deep, deep breath, and exhale slowly. I do that once or twice. The process immediately helps me regain control of what might otherwise progress into a runaway adrenaline response. Obviously, do not close your eyes to do this if you are driving. That would *not* be a good way to reduce stress! Your longer session will work well in the morning or before meals.

Sit Comfortably

Choose a quiet environment where you will not be disturbed. Wear loose-fitting, comfortable clothing, and find a sitting position that feels good to you. Some people opt for a straight-backed chair; others sit in the classic position, cross-legged on the floor. Your spine should be vertical, your shoulders relaxed, your arms resting comfortably on your thighs or at your sides, your jaw relaxed and open slightly, and your eyes closed. The goal is comfort, but you should also sit with a sense of pride and confidence. Many beginning meditators feel silly trying to sit a certain way. The most important thing is that you sit your own way, the way in which you feel good about yourself, however that may be.

Breathing Is Key

All meditation is rooted in proper breathing. Studies have shown that many of us simply do not fill our lungs deeply enough and that we actually reduce our oxygen intake during periods of stress. The techniques you learn and develop during meditation may help you breathe more effectively at other times during the day when stress is high.

Relaxed, deep, therapeutic breathing comes from the abdomen. This type of breathing, also called belly breathing, makes full and more effective use of your diaphragm, the muscular membrane that forms a floor underneath the lungs. When you breathe normally your diaphragm relaxes and contracts. When you "breathe with your belly" it expands even more so, allowing the lungs to fill with more air.

To begin, inhale through your nose (unless it is stuffy from allergies or a cold) and try to relax your belly. When you inhale, your belly should naturally expand outward as your diaphragm pushes down, and the air should flow freely in and out. As nourishing oxygen flows into your lungs, the nooks and crannies of the lungs' air sacs that are closed with shallow respirations open and inflate and move life-sustaining oxygen into your bloodstream. When you exhale through your mouth, pull in your belly to fully expel air. With each expulsion of air you are expelling carbon dioxide and other "exhaust" from your body's metabolic processes. Overall, your cycle of breathing should become slower and deeper.

Practicing Transcendental Meditation

All meditation features a point of focus to calm your mind and prevent distracting thoughts. If you practice TM, you will use a mantra to achieve this. Pick a relaxing word (you may have heard of *om* as a commonly used mantra). Repeat it silently. If you decide to take a meditation class, your instructor may provide a different Sanskrit sound to repeat, such as *kirim* or *aheim*. If such sounds don't work for you, remember the Benson adaptation of TM and repeat any word or phrase that has meaning for you. I personally find that using a mantra, devoid of any association, allows me to shut down distracting thoughts.

Try to maintain a passive attitude. When distracting events or thoughts enter your mind, do not focus on them or try to push them out of your awareness. Simply let them float in and then out again, always returning to your mantra. For instance, if a siren catches your attention as you are meditating, you may begin to visualize a police car. The noise may make you feel annoyed or tense. Your mind will start to get excited. Just notice the sensations. Let them come and go. Let the siren go. Continue to breathe deeply, and repeat your mantra as you do so.

If you are just beginning to practice meditation, you may feel frustrated and find that you are very easily distracted and somewhat self-conscious. These are normal feelings. Remember that maintaining focus takes practice.

You may also feel as though you do not have time for the luxury of meditation. Just remember: You are reading this book because you have realized that you need to become less stressed. If you keep repeating the same patterns and expect things to change, you are setting yourself up for failure. There is almost nothing more important than taking time out from your hectic day to quiet your busy mind and give it a rest.

Practicing Awareness Meditation

As I explained earlier, awareness, or mindful meditation can also induce a state of deep relaxation. But its practitioners view it as more than just a stress reduction technique. The goal of mindfulness is to become aware and in touch with your life in the present moment.

Mindful meditation teaches an exercise called sitting meditation, which begins with the same sitting posture and deep breathing used in TM. When you breathe, do not focus on your breath so much that you consciously control it; simply become aware that you are breathing. This awareness is your focal point. As you meditate, thoughts or feelings may pop into your mind. Do not view them as distractions. Rather, witness them passively and nonjudgmentally as events in the field of your awareness. In this way you take a step back from your thoughts and are less likely to take them so personally, which makes them less likely to arouse stress responses. As your thoughts recede, return to the awareness of your breath. In this way, mindful meditation is simply a process of fine-tuning your moment-to-moment awareness.

Mini Meditation

Throughout the day, I recommend that you take several short breaks to relax, breathe, and reenergize. In this way you can recenter yourself and dissolve stress as it occurs. You can keep your eyes open or closed, depending on where you are and your comfort level. You may choose to add a silent mantra to your breathing, much as in your longer meditation session.

Try setting this book down right now and take in several deep, diaphragmatic breaths. There is no time like the present to begin to practice the techniques that will help you live a healthier and more robust life.

How Will You Feel after Meditating?

At the end of a successful TM or mindfulness session, you should feel alert, energized, and in control of your emotions. I personally can attest that meditation is extremely rejuvenating. As a busy physician, I have a very stressful lifestyle and need to use these techniques regularly to maintain my high energy and positive outlook. My patients who practice meditation techniques tell me that they feel the same way. They report that meditation is one of their most useful life skills because it keeps things in perspective and allows them to experience a greater sense of control over their lives.

What about a Class?

The fact that mindful meditation has so many component practices underscores the need for proper instruction. The basics of all meditation forms can be self-taught. But if you are serious about practicing meditation because you face severe stress or suffer serious health problems, you should invest in a formal meditation-training program. Trained experts have refined meditation techniques that offer the most benefits. A good instructor can guide you and help you learn properly so you practice correctly and most effectively. Transcendental meditation classes are quite common in many communities, as are mindfulness-based stress reduction (MBSR) programs.

Progressive Relaxation

Systematically tensing and relaxing various parts of your body also has been shown to effectively help your mind and body relax.

To practice this technique, you can either sit in a relaxed position or lie down comfortably. Soft music playing in the background can help distract you from other noises in your environment.

Begin by breathing deeply, using the diaphragm fully, in and out. As you start to inhale again, slowly curl your toes as tightly as you can and hold that position until you need to exhale. As you begin to exhale, allow your toes to relax to their normal positions. Repeat this toe-tensing exercise two more times. Then move to the arch of the foot, using the same tense-relax process. Progressively move up the legs, then the arms, then the hips, waist, abdomen, chest, neck, face, and scalp. When you are done, you may feel as if you have had a full-body massage. In effect, you have.

Mindful meditation teaches a similar practice, in which you "check in" with your body and remind yourself to exist in the present moment. In these moments become aware of your slower, deeper breathing, and let your thoughts come and go. You might also perform a "body scan" by systematically focusing your attention on the various regions of your body, feet to head. When you do this, note any physical sensations you are experiencing in those parts of your body. When performed as a more formal process while the patient is lying down, the body scan process helps people cope with chronic pain and other physical problems.

Emergency Stress Relief

Stress can sometimes come on so quickly that emergency measures are required. Bill Crawford, Ph.D., a counselor and lecturer in Houston, Texas, has developed a method for dealing with stress emergencies.

Crawford believes stress to be the result of a chemical reaction caused by five components:

1. Feelings of being out of control
2. Feelings of tension
3. Negative self-talk or complaining
4. Worry about what is going to happen next
5. Negative responses such as fear, anger, fatigue, and frustration

A chain reaction of stress can take place in a matter of seconds, says Crawford. This triggers the primitive part of our brain to react, often in the negative ways that I have outlined in previous chapters. Rapid changes in neurotransmitters, the chemicals that carry signals between the different parts of the brain, can occur in an instant to prepare us either for battle or retreat.

To prevent or calm a fight-or-flight reaction, Crawford recommends using techniques that can be remembered by the acronym BRAIN:

1. **Breathe.**
2. **Relax.**
3. **Ask, "How would I rather be feeling?"**
4. **Imagine feeling that.**
5. **Notice the change.**

Breathe

As soon as you start to feel out of control, take three to five deep breaths. Doing this gives you two advantages, says Crawford. First, it gives you a short break and keeps you from acting without thinking, as many people tend to do in stressful situations. It also allows the more evolved, thinking part of your brain—the neocortex—to gain control. Crawford believes that taking a break to breathe will help you to respond to stress in a more purposeful way.

Relax

Another physical response to stress is muscle tension. According to Crawford, fatigue often hits in a stress situation because a person has to fight tense muscles just to function.

"I encourage people to pair their breathing with the word *relax*," says Crawford. "If you say it when you exhale, it works almost like a command to the muscles of your body."

Ask, "How Would I Rather Be Feeling?"

Negative self-talk is almost always a part of the stress cycle, says Crawford. You start to ask, "What is wrong with me?" or "What is wrong with that person?" That kind of thinking leads to negative feelings about yourself and others, which leads to more stress.

Instead of asking those kinds of rhetorical questions Crawford suggests asking yourself this one, simple question: "How would I rather be feeling?"

The answers, says Crawford, will usually be feelings such as: calm, confident, in control, and serene.

"You can begin to call up any of these feelings just by thinking about them," says Crawford. "Those feelings are there if you ask for them."

Imagine Feeling That

Next, says Crawford, imagine feeling the way you want to feel. If you would like to feel calm, imagine a time in the past when you felt that way. The same goes for other feelings, such as feeling in control, powerful, or content.

"The problem to overcome is that most of us were taught to worry by the people who love us," Crawford explains. "When you were a kid, your mom always told you to be careful when you went out to play. This translated as, 'Worry about bad things happening in order to be safe.' Now we have to overcome that part of us that says worry will keep us safe. What it will really do is make us sick."

Notice the Change

Finally, take time to notice the changes that these simple thought exercises have produced. If you have done them correctly, you will have changed a stressful reaction to a soothing one, says Crawford, because you have inspired your brain to produce calming chemicals instead of stressful ones.

Further, you will now be in a position to choose a more purposeful response.

I think using BRAIN is especially effective in emergency situations in which stress sneaks up on you quickly. It gives you an easy-to-remember package of tools that you can grab and use.

Crawford believes that we can actually change the chemical makeup of our bodies by following this model. Instead of producing the chemicals of stress, you can teach your body to produce chemicals more congruent with how you want to feel. This mind-body interaction has been proven over and over again.

Stress Reduction Techniques and Your Health

Whatever technique you choose, you should take the attitude that stress reduction is a necessary survival technique. It is good mind-body hygiene—like a daily mental bath or shower—not a luxury for a privileged few or the health obsessed.

A growing number of individuals, researchers, and health care providers are coming to realize that meditation and similar forms of relaxation can lead to better health, higher quality of life, and lowered health care costs. Most important, meditation techniques offer the potential for learning how to live in an increasingly complex and stressful society while helping to preserve health in the process.

Stress Management Techniques and Cardiovascular Health

A recent Duke University Medical Center study found that heart disease patients who learn how to manage their stress are 77% less likely to have a heart attack or require cardiac surgery than patients who receive only standard medical care. These patients practiced aerobics for 35 minutes three times per week, or participated in a weekly stress management program that taught them how to reduce stress through relaxation and how to change their responses to stressful events.

A study by the College of Maharishi Vedic Medicine (in Iowa) found that transcendental meditation (TM) provided impressive cardiovascular benefits that could help people avoid a heart attack or stroke. The study monitored 60 African-American men and women with high blood pressure. One group of subjects practiced TM for 20 minutes twice a day, and the other participated in a health education program. The TM group experienced significant decline in the thickness of the wall of the carotid artery, allowing it to carry more blood to the brain. The group that practiced meditation also showed a greater decrease in blood pressure and heart rate.

Another study at the College of Maharishi Vedic Medicine documented a decrease in free radical activity (which contributes to atherosclerosis) after subjects participated in a meditation program.

Stress Management Techniques and Women's Health

Stress reduction may help infertile women conceive. Researchers at New England Deaconness Hospital in Boston had 54 women who were having difficulty becoming pregnant undergo a behavioral treatment program that included meditation. In addition to showing a significant decrease in anxiety, depression, and fatigue, 34% of these women became pregnant within six months of completing the study.

Meditation may have other benefits for women. Researchers at Harvard Medical School found that women experienced a significant decrease in physical symptoms associated with PMS after three months of daily meditation.

Psychological Benefits of Meditation

Apart from easing conditions and preventing disease, meditation seems to make its practitioners more psychologically and physiologically stable, less anxious, and more able to experience a sense of control in their lives. A study at the University of California found that people who practice mindful meditation, which emphasizes detached observation and awareness, experienced fewer psychological problems, a greater sense of control in their lives, and more meaningful spiritual experiences than those who did not meditate. Researchers concluded that meditation may transform the way we deal with life events.

CHAPTER EIGHT

Step 4: Rekindling Relationships

Conditions at home and in the workplace are among the greatest contributors to female stress. That these two elements of a person's life contribute so greatly to stress should be no surprise. After all, work and family occupy most of our waking hours.

Some studies show that women are more likely to experience stress at home and in the workplace when they feel as though they have little control over their surroundings and circumstances. For instance, organizations that are poorly run and don't allow employee involvement in the decision-making process have more stressed employees. The same is true at home: A woman who feels as though her husband is unsympathetic is likely to feel stressed in her home environment.

Many of my patients are experiencing relationship problems that are the result of what is going on inside of them as well as outside. But after a few weeks of taking DHEA, they are able to tell the difference between those problems that are the result of hormonal imbalances and those caused by interpersonal friction.

However, sometimes we manufacture our own stress in the way we respond to events. We may overrespond, becoming stressed about things that don't warrant such extreme reactions.

Whole books have been written filled with helpful advice on how to manage your relationships in every aspect of your life—at work, with your children, parents, friends, siblings, and so forth. Here we'll focus on what my experience has shown to be one of the most significant ways of reducing the stress in your life: enhancing your relationship with your spouse, partner, or significant other.

The "Stressful" You vs. The "Unstressful" You

Elaine brought her husband, Tony, with her to our appointment to evaluate her stress-related complaints. He seemed very angry as she recited the litany of complaints that define female stress (fatigue, depression, weight gain, irritability, etc.). But he literally turned crimson when she told me that she was no longer interested in sex and that she was tired of virtually everything in her life.

"Tony," I said. "Do you want to say anything?"

"Yes," he said, glaring at his wife. "Maybe I'm tired of a few things, too."

He fell silent again as Elaine described him as "unsympathetic" and "self-centered," but he looked as if he was going to explode. Clearly, this couple needed to work on their relationship as part of Elaine's stress reduction program.

I explained the biological basis for stress to Elaine and Tony, and then I drew some blood. I started Elaine on DHEA supplements. During her next few visits, I added vitamin supplements and an exercise program.

A few months later Elaine came back a new woman, energized and filled with enthusiasm about life. She told me she had regained her good humor and had a newfound interest in sex.

She had one problem left, though.

"My husband is still reacting to the 'stressful' me," she said. "I understand why he feels this way, but I don't know what to do. Is there a way I can repair our relationship?"

I have seen this happen many times. I prescribe DHEA and lifestyle changes, and my patient becomes her old, unstressed self in a very short period of time. But although her significant other has probably been hoping to see that unstressed self for some time, he or she may have difficulty reconnecting with that new persona. As a result, many couples become frustrated in their relationships once the patient's stress has been relieved.

When this happens I usually explain that these problems often can be overcome with a little nurturing. I present them with this list of 30 practical suggestions for nurturing a relationship that has been victimized by stress.

Share these with your spouse or partner, and try to implement them in your own relationship on a routine basis. They are simple but effective ways to heal emotional wounds.

Thirty Ways to Keep Your Lover

1. DATE NIGHT   Establishing (and keeping to!) a date night can keep the fires burning in a relationship and provide perspective in the midst of a life that can sometimes feel more like a crazy war.

My wife and I have been practicing date night for three years. It is the highlight of our week, and it has been a great way to reduce stress and help us reconnect. We get together each and every Wednesday, with no exceptions. This is sacred time that is meant for just the two of us. We chose Wednesdays because we felt that day provided a much-needed midweek break from the routines of work, cooking, cleaning, and child rearing, and from the mounting stresses and fraying patience that went along with them.

Frequently dinner and a movie provide the perfect escape. If funds are short, however, we'll grab a quick snack and take a nice stroll. The key is that no other people are involved; date night is for just the two of us.

2. THE DAILY MILE   A great way to relieve stress and connect at the same time is through mutual activity. Walking together offers a chance to catch up on the day's activities in a neutral setting. Not only is this good for the body, it is also good for the mind and soul.

I have found that some of the most frustrating moments in my day will dissipate after just a few minutes of brisk walking. Getting out for a daily fitness walk can help clear out the stale air, so to speak. This can be a great way to erase the mental agenda that keeps many women from getting a good night's sleep. And that's not even to mention the physical benefits of this wonderful form of exercise!

3. SHOWER TOGETHER   Time spent together in the shower can be a refreshing way to feel alive and connected. Warm water is soothing to the body, mind, and soul. Showers wash off the stress of daily life, allowing worries to flow down the drain. Just the mutual washing of each other's backs can help remind partners that there are things in life more meaningful than work and bills. So do your part for water conservation and hit the showers together. It's good clean fun!

4. TUB TIME   Do you prefer the tub to the shower? Break out the bubble bath and jump in. It is virtually impossible to keep stress and tension alive in a warm tub. Take time to relax and talk amongst the suds. Experience the warmth of the water and the closeness of your partner. Sit facing each other and give each other a simultaneous foot and calf rub. Or you can take turns sitting back to front, trading other nice, slippery, soothing back and shoulder massages. Whichever position you choose, don't rush to get clean. Let the warmth of the water sooth those tired muscles. Enjoy the closeness of your partner.

5. MASSAGE YOUR MATE   A loving massage is a stress-reducing activity you can both enjoy, whether you are on the giving or receiving end.

Use some warm, lightly scented oil and begin with the small of the back, where much tension is focused. Allow the warm oil to soak in as you gently apply enough pressure to feel the muscles relax. Use circular and repetitive motions.

As you give the massage, notice that your tension flows down and out of your arms. If you are the recipient, feel the stress leave your body with every soothing stroke.

You don't need to take a class to become an expert at this stress reducer. All you need is time, a little warm massage oil, and a willing partner. Add some calming music and a candle or two, and feel the tension melt away.

6. LET THE MUSIC TAKE YOU   Music has always been a great way to diffuse stress. But did you know that it can also be a great way to reconnect and strengthen a relationship? Attending a music event such as a free concert, live band, or a popular artist can help the two of you unwind after even the most stressful day. Seeing a concert by a popular artist is usually worth the long wait in line, just to experience the magnitude of energy that emanates from such performances.

Listening to any kind of music together at home can be very soothing and can help push away the worries of the day and allow the more important feelings of passion and unity to come through. There are also many products specifically for stress reduction available on CD, DVD, and audiocassette that can be played anywhere to stimulate the senses and calm the nerves.

7. DO SOMETHING EXTRAORDINARY   Get out of the routine, break out of the mold, shake it up. Go to a new store, sleep on opposite sides of the bed, change places at dinner. Routines can be good, but breaking them can be even better. If you always say "no," try saying "yes!" If you are a "yes" person, say "no" once in a while. Spontaneity can be the spice of life, and it can be a path out of the predictable boredom many relationships fall prey to. Breaking free can be a first step in decreasing your stress response.

8. GO TO A COMEDY SHOW   We often find ourselves locked in a perpetually gloomy state. When that happens, it may take a professional to help us out—a professional comic, that is!

Laughing together can be very beneficial for couples. When you laugh, your brain is flooded with feel-good neurotransmitters, and many of the overwhelming thoughts are chased right out of your consciousness.

So go to a comedy show . . . but be prepared to let yourself go. Laughing out loud can happen only when your inhibitions have been overcome.

9. TAKE OUT A BOARD GAME   Get the family together to play a board game. Games like Monopoly, Clue, Pictionary, Cranium, and Yahtzee take little effort to set up and play, and they will all turn down your stress meter. Card games are also great stress reducers.

Games are what I call structured-unstructured activities, in which daily stresses evaporate and are replaced by newer, less critical ones, such as "Do I have enough money to buy Boardwalk and Park Place?"

10. TAKE A NATURE WALK   Nature has a unique way of reminding you of your priorities. It helps to ground you when you feel that the world is turning too fast. Clear your mind by listening to the sounds of nature. Breathe deeply and let the stress and tension leave your body as fresh air enters. With it will come a sense that all is right with your world.

11. DO SOMETHING FOR OTHERS   Giving back is yet another way to renew the bond between you. Doing for others not only benefits the recipients of your good deeds, but it is also good for your relationship. Helping people less fortunate than yourselves can make your own cares and worries seem less overwhelming. Performing such an activity together may bring out a caring side in each of you that you may not have seen when you were each wrapped up in your own "stress shells." Seeing each other give freely and sharing that gift together can help remind you of the value of togetherness and the power of two hearts beating as one.

12. DEVELOP A HOBBY TOGETHER   Couples can learn a hobby like golf, tennis, or racquetball and get their exercise at the same time. I have several friends who take dance lessons together as a break from their regular routines. Others snow ski together, and some of their most treasured experiences are from these trips. Couples can enjoy arts and crafts activities together. Or they can indulge in antique shopping. Whatever fits your fancy, a hobby can be an enjoyable experience that strengthens your bond and gives both of you a focal point for your time and energy.

Experiment until you find a hobby that both of you can enjoy. It should be fulfilling and interesting enough to commit your time and energy to. It should be equally enjoyable for both of you and should be something that each of you can excel at if you so desire. A recent 10-year study confirmed that "serious leisure" like a hobby or an activity that involves your whole being was the best guarantee of long-term happiness. Interestingly, dancing ranked at the top of the list.

13. TAKE A DAY TO PLAY   Sometimes we all need to take a mental health day off from work and just play. Taking an unscheduled day to be together and share the joy of not following a schedule can go a long way toward restoring passion and romance that tend to get squelched by the pressures of life. Recognizing that your relationship is the priority and can take center stage once in a while can help you reaffirm where the priorities in your life really stand.

Are there places in your city you have always wanted to explore? Are there local sights you haven't had time to see? What activities have the two of you wanted to do but haven't because you've been too stressed out or busy to do them? Use this day to change the pattern from work first, then play, to play all day!

Caution: Resist the temptation to stay home and do all the chores that have been piling up. Take the day and get out and *enjoy yourselves.*

14. TAKE A CLASS TOGETHER   Find a topic of mutual interest, and take the class as a couple. The time spent together may be a great diversion from the routines you have established, and the topic may also help to get your mind off your usual thoughts. Learning new ideas and thoughts are good ways to keep the brain active and continue expanding our life experience. Some classes stimulate further conversation on the way home or at a café over a cup of your favorite beverage.

Colleges, universities, community centers, churches, and civic groups all have classes to offer. Many are free or inexpensive and cover a range of topics, from arts and activities to yoga, massage, and psychology.

15. GO TO THE LIBRARY   Browse through the topics, and stop when something piques your interest. Show it to your partner and then go on to something new. Experience the moment. Allow new information to bombard your senses, and block out the stress gremlins that compete for your every thought. You may discover new interests or revive dormant ones—and your partner will be learning more about you.

If you let them, libraries can bring back old memories. Many of us have long forgotten their smells and sounds. Take some time to sit down to review some of the books you couldn't put down as a college student. Read something you have wanted to read but never had the time. Look at books that show you other places in the world, and think about the magnitude of the universe. Are our problems really so big? Or have we just lost some perspective? Enjoy the moment with your partner and absorb the tranquility that libraries foster. Take some of this tranquility with you as you leave, and savor it at those times when stress threatens.

16. CAMP OUT IN YOUR LIVING ROOM   Make a tent out of bedspreads, or blow up an air mattress. Throw the couch cushions on the floor and use only flashlights. Bring your favorite snacks and hide under the covers. Turn out all the lights and "rough it" for the night. If you have a fireplace, get it started and feel the warmth of natural heat. Drink hot chocolate.

"Remember when" is a great game to play when you are house camping. Review those great times and relive fond memories. Reminisce about old times when your life was simpler, and consider ways in which you can get there again.

Look at the ceiling, not at the cobwebs. Your home has a different perspective from this position.

Enjoy the simplicity of the moment and the opportunity to slow down. Did you remember to take the phone off the hook, campers?

17. TAKE A BUS RIDE   A novel activity to experience together is to take a bus ride around the city in which you live. If you routinely drive to work and do not take the bus, this can be especially adventurous. Taking a bus ride with no destination allows you to experience the pace from the grandstand. As you ride, look out the window and observe the people on the sidewalks. What do you see? Ponder some of these questions: Who is going where, and what for? Are they fulfilled? Are they stressed? What is important? Why do I do what I do? Am I doing what is important? Are we really enjoying ourselves or is this all we know how to do? These are questions I have pondered when I have taken existential rides through my city of Seattle. Take the time to interact with your partner about the feelings that have been awakened by these few moments of being a spectator rather than a participant in life.

18. TAKE THE TRAIN   Taking a train to another town can be an inexpensive and enjoyable excursion. The rhythmic clattering of the railroad tracks sets the cadence for a peaceful escape from the current reality. Such a classic form of transportation allows you to enjoy traveling *through* the landscape rather than *over* it, as you do when traveling by plane. Take advantage of the fact that you aren't the one doing the driving! Look out the window and notice the gradual changes in scenery. Enjoy the sensation of the world flying past as you sit in comfort, letting the steady movement relax you. Don't forget to take pleasure in each other's company as you both unwind. All aboard!

19. ESCAPE FOR A WEEKEND   Load up an overnight bag and let the spirit of adventure take you away for a while. Don't bother to plan. Many times we are so scheduled that the schedule itself becomes a stressor. Instead, throw deadlines and time pressures out the window as you head off for your escape. Maybe you won't make it any farther than just across town. When you get to wherever you are going, stay up as late as you want and sleep in the next morning. This treat can be particularly wonderful after you have just completed a long project or been through a period of intense stress.

20. CATCH UP WITH FRIENDS   We frequently give so many hours to our work and work-related activities that we have little time left for other priorities, like close friends. The old adage "When you are on your deathbed you won't wish you had spent more time at the office" is very true. Is there someone you wish you spent more time with? Compose a letter, make a phone call, or schedule a visit. By nurturing outside relationships, couples' relationships can be enhanced.

21. WRITE A LOVE LETTER   Do you remember when you would write letters to your loved one? Letters can restore our sense of accurate communication. They allow us to present a point of view without interruption and can at times be a better form of communication than oral argument. In conversations it is easy to remember only the hurtful comments and not the positive ones. In letters the good comments are recorded forever in black and white. Your partner can read your loving words over and over again.

22. SHARE FIVE POSITIVES   We rarely take the time to tell those closest to us just how much we appreciate their good qualities. Why not tell your partner how much he or she is doing right for you, and how much you appreciate it?

Give yourselves 20 minutes to write down five positive qualities about each other. Try to be as specific as possible. For instance, if you list honesty for your partner, give several examples of when he or she has exhibited that quality, or why being honest is important to you and how it makes you feel when your partner is honest.

This exercise allows us to refocus on the very best qualities in our partners. It also allows us also to look at ourselves in a positive light. When your partner reads you his or her list, enjoy the feedback and let those comments overtake any negative feelings you have about yourself. Savor the moment.

23. ASK FOR AND OFFER   There is something to be said for accepting each other as we are, but there is also benefit in trying to satisfy each other's needs in the relationship. We all have behaviors that can be annoying. We can usually change some of these quite easily if we are made aware of the effect they have on our mates.

Make a list of requests or behaviors that you would like your partner to try to improve, and ask him or her to do the same for you. If this exercise is undertaken from a loving point of view and you can share each list without becoming defensive, then your relationship may become much more fruitful and fulfilling. This activity can be a very loving and caring gesture that goes a great distance in developing mutual respect for your relationship. Compromise can be a real energy producer.

24. LET'S MAKE A DEAL   There are certain things that you wish your spouse would do for you, and most likely there are also things you could do in return. Why not negotiate to fulfill each other's requests? Has the garage been looking like a disaster area lately? Are there too many magazines lying around the house? Whatever the request, set aside some time to address these tasks. The two of you can actually have fun and complete things that have been on the to-do list for an extended period of time.

25. TAKE TIME TO TALK   A thriving relationship needs quality time to be sustained. But quality time must also go hand in hand with a certain quantity of time to avoid the deterioration of a healthy relationship. Decreased interest in each other—decreased interest in sex, decreased energy, and decreased commitment—can also occur when one person in a relationship does not devote enough time to his or her mate. If this occurs day after day, resentment and defensiveness will grow, eventually spoiling the time you do have with each other.

Lack of time spent together is one of the most common reasons for separation and divorce. Do not underestimate the value of both quantity and quality time when it comes to your relationship.

26. PRACTICE ACTIVE LISTENING   People usually want to be listened to without interruption or comment. When your partner is talking, try to just listen. Resist the temptation to justify or defend yourself, and take the time to make sure you understand the real message behind what the other person is saying. When the person is done speaking, you can practice active listening by reflecting back what he or she has said with comments such as: "It sounds like you feel as though . . . ," or "I get the feeling you are really worried about . . ."

Once you have mastered the skill of active listening without becoming defensive and developed the ability to ask questions without being threatening, you will feel safe communicating with your partner at a deep and devoted level. Taking time to talk can be the very foundation of keeping your relationship healthy and strong.

27. RELAX AND REVIEW   Parks are wonderful settings for helping you to slow down. Watching others share relaxed meals with friends, families, and loved ones, as you do the same with your partner, can help reassure you that it is all right for you to take some down time once in a while, too. Use this time to discuss the important qualities of your relationship and to work on those that may need buffing up. Here is some material to use in your discussion:

Researchers note that there are 10 factors that make a relationship work: faithfulness and loyalty to your partner; mutual respect and appreciation; understanding and tolerance; not wanting a partner to change; having a fulfilling sexual relationship; talking openly and communicating; sharing common interests; expressing emotions; sharing chores; and having independent interests.

Taking the time to discuss these items as you and your partner share a picnic in a beautiful, natural setting will help you put your stresses in perspective and reset your priorities.

28. HELP YOURSELF TO SELF-HELP   Remember that relationships need care and attention, especially under periods of intense stress and pressure. It can be very productive to take a little time each night to sit with your partner, read a passage from one of these books, and see how the two of you could incorporate the advice into your relationship. Use the books as starting points for discussion. It can be refreshing to know that you are the not only ones who have gone through this type of situation and that there is a lot of hope for getting you back on track if you're having problems. Read, discuss, and learn. What strategies may fit? What can the two of you do to increase the pleasure you get from each other?

29. SEEK PROFESSIONAL HELP   Don't be afraid to see a professional therapist or counselor if you are having difficulty in your relationship. Stress can be extremely taxing on a relationship and can color the perspectives of both parties. A professional counselor can help restore perspectives that may be more appropriate and constructive than your current ones.

As the tension created by stress and overwhelming responsibilities mount and DHEA stores become depleted, our perceptions can be altered to the point of complete dysfunction. It can become next to impossible to resurrect a relationship on your own when things have been out of control for too long. It is not a sign of weakness to ask for help from a trusted professional to help get things back on track. Professionals are skilled in keeping communication open and helping each person understand the meaning behind words, which can be easily misinterpreted if anger and defensiveness get in the way. A good referee can help restore communication between couples who have lost their way.

Usually the techniques learned in therapy sessions are easily worked into your daily routine, and couples come away from counseling with new coping skills. In addition, a skilled counselor can help you learn not only which elements in your relationship trigger your stress response, but also which behaviors you can use as a force field to prevent that response from taking place.

30. FORGIVE YOURSELF   You may feel guilty or angry with yourself for the way you have acted toward your loved ones as you have suffered through the trials of female stress. My advice is to resist these feelings. Most of your problems were caused by elements out of your control, that is, human physiology. As your DHEA levels dropped, so did your ability to handle the stresses of life. Now that you are taking DHEA and your life is returning to normal, you are free of the emotional and physical bonds of female stress. Rejoice in that freedom. Forgive, forget, and move on.

CHAPTER NINE

Step 5: Effective Exercising

As we go about our daily activities—work, child care, errands, chores—we often begin to feel more and more tightly wound, as though there were some sort of anxiety spring inside of us. At some point during the day we need to do something to unwind the spring and release the tension. An excellent way to do this is through exercise.

In this chapter I will explain how exercise works to relieve stress and enhance health. Then I will show you how to begin an exercise program that can become a regular and enjoyable part of your life. Before long you will wonder how you ever got along without it.

The Exercise Contradiction

How exercise relieves stress can be difficult to understand, since, paradoxically, exercise brings about many of the physiologic changes brought on by stress itself. Yet exercise does eliminate—and even prevent—feelings of stress.

Here is how that happens.

When you exercise, your body goes through the following changes:

- Your neurotransmitters fire up
- Hormones—including cortisol—flood your body

- Your heart races
- Your breathing speeds up
- Your blood pressure rises
- Your muscles tense
- You become focused

These are all the responses that a woman experiences during a fight-or-flight reaction to a stressful situation. So why is exercise any better than just plain stress? Modern stress prepares you for a fight or flight that doesn't come.

When we experience stress, all of the physiologic reactions previously mentioned take place; yet none of the products of these reactions get used.

The brain becomes bathed in stress chemicals that aren't expended. The body becomes flooded with hormones, like cortisol, that continue to circulate in the bloodstream. Blood pressure rises, and muscles tense in anticipation of a physical confrontation that doesn't take place. Exercise utilizes the products of all that stress, providing an outlet for the pressure of your day's stresses and making it possible for you to feel calm once your workout is over.

Another benefit of exercises like bicycling, jogging, or cross-country skiing is that they require consistent repetitive motion that has a similar effect on the brain as meditation. The repetitive breathing and movement required in these "moving meditation" exercises help to soothe your nerves and inspire calmness and tranquility. In some ways, Friedrich Nietzsche, the German philosopher, summed up the effects of exercise best when he said, "A few hours of mountain climbing turn a rascal and a saint into two pretty similar creatures."

A rascal who turned into a saint in my own practice is a woman I'll call Barb. A slim woman with a constant frown on her face, Barb came to see me because she had heard that I had "something" that could improve her disposition. Everything seemed to be going wrong in her life, Barb told me, even though nothing had really changed. Her husband had worked at the same job for years, and her children were doing "respectable work" in school and not getting into trouble. She, on the other hand, had turned into a "hot reactor," someone who became angry over the smallest things.

Barb was nearing 40 years of age, and I could tell by looking at her that she might be headed for an early menopause. Still, her DHEA levels were well within the acceptable levels. What should I do?

"We are going to start conservatively," I told Barb. Instead of prescribing DHEA, I suggested a few lifestyle changes to see what effect those might have on her. I instructed her to drink less coffee, get more sleep, and perform half an hour of exercise daily.

At first she wasn't happy with just a lifestyle prescription. Like most patients, she wanted some kind of magic pill to get rid of her problem. When she came back two weeks later, however, Barb was very pleased to have learned that something as simple as a morning walk could eliminate her problem. What she said summed up the one aspect of exercise that is too often ignored. "I had forgotten how pleasant working out can be. It takes the edge off every problem or thought I have."

Exercise and Weight Loss

One of the major benefits of exercise is that it increases your metabolism, the rate at which your body burns calories. We all know people who can eat as many sweets and high-fat foods as they want and not gain an ounce. Most likely, those people have high metabolisms. They are also probably less likely to convert the energy they get from food into fat. The good news is, you don't have to be born with this type of predisposition. By exercising, you can significantly step up your metabolism.

After a vigorous aerobic workout, your metabolic rate jumps 25% for up to 15 hours afterward, allowing you to burn calories more quickly. In addition, your workout speeds up your digestive process, causing you to absorb fewer calories.

In addition to boosting your metabolism, physical activity helps reduce body fat. Researchers at the Washington University School of Medicine found that sedentary menopausal women carried 13% more body fat than fit menopausal women.

Excess fat also places stress on your ligaments, tendons, bones, and muscles. Liza, a longtime patient of mine, came to see me for her annual pelvic exam and Pap smear. She limped into the examining room, put on a gown, and managed to get herself up onto the examining table. But when she tried to get her feet into the stirrups, she found it was impossible. "I fell last week and reinjured my knee," she said to the medical assistant. "I'm only 35, but I feel a lot older." The she recited a list of blood pressure medications she was taking.

Liza's knee injury was so severe, and her leg so swollen, that we had to cancel the Pap smear and focus on her knee instead. It gave me a prime opportunity to talk to her about her weight problem.

I asked Liza how many times she had tried to lose weight.

"Dr. Vern, I have tried just about every diet I have read about or seen on TV. I have been to a bunch of commercial weight loss centers and groups. Nothing has worked, and I am just too tired to fight it anymore. I have given up hope. Each time I begin a diet I think I have the willpower to follow it, but I just keep inching up on the scale. I don't exactly know how much I weigh because our home scale only goes to 300 pounds," she said, taking a very deep breath and letting it out on a prolonged sigh.

Liza was dressed perfectly, in vibrant colors that reflected her dynamic personality, but I could see the real woman behind the bright colors. She was a tired, frustrated, hardworking, attractive, 316-pound woman lost in a body twice as large as it should have been for good health.

I had a long discussion with Liza about obesity. I explained that it was already having a serious effect on her health. Obviously, the trendy diets she was trying had not been helping her. I promised to give her some suggestions and basic lifestyle improvement tips, all baby steps that she could easily follow on the path to becoming a healthier person.

Perhaps the most important of those was a regular program of exercise.

"My grandfather used to say that it is as easy to develop good habits as it is to develop bad ones," I told her. I have learned in my career that this is very true. People can do amazing things, if started at a pace they can succeed at. New exercise habits must be introduced in small and incremental steps. I cannot stress how important that is.

I asked Liza to begin a walking program, starting with only short distances. I told her I would prefer she go to the mailbox and back if that was all she could do—as long as she did something. When she saw that she could conquer this short distance, she would perceive it as a success. Then she could increase the distance a little until she could tolerate that, as well.

She would need this series of small successes as positive reinforcements to help her develop her new exercise habit.

Liza was excited for the first time in years. She was going to adopt simple lifestyle changes and a new habit of exercise to replace her old weight-gaining lifestyle.

Exercise and Bone Health

Weight-bearing activities like walking or stair climbing, and strength-training exercises are all recommended for maintaining stronger bones. This is necessary because as you age your bones naturally lose their mineral content. During the first five to 10 years after menopause, the average bone loss is 2%. By age 60 you could easily lose 15–30% of your bone mass. How does it happen?

When your ovaries stop producing estrogen, which helps deposit and maintain calcium in the bones, you experience 3–5% bone erosion per year for several years. This weakens the internal supporting structure of your bones, making them more prone to fracturing. This disorder is called osteoporosis.

Increasing calcium in your diet may help increase bone mass, but calcium and calcium supplements alone may not stop bone loss entirely. And while fluoride has been proven to increase bone mass by up to 10%, it has not been shown to prevent fractures related to osteoporosis. Estrogen replacement therapy can reduce the likelihood of bone fractures by 70%, but for many women it has negative side effects.

Exercise is a proven bone booster, and it has no negative side effects. New evidence shows that weight-bearing exercise such as walking and jogging significantly increases bone mass. In a study of postmenopausal women at the State University of New York at Buffalo School of Medicine, researchers found that women who walked one hour more than other women had thicker, stronger bones in their hips than sedentary women. In fact, their bone mass equaled that of women four years younger. In another study of more than 200 postmenopausal women, those who walked 7.5 miles per week had a higher average bone mass density than those who walked less than one mile each week.

Your bones are never too old to benefit from an exercise program. Researchers at the Washington University School of Medicine found that women aged 55–70 who did walking, jogging, and stair climbing increased their bone mass by about 6%, while inactive women of comparable ages showed no increase.

Exercise and Muscle Mass

Exercise also helps you maintain your muscle mass as you age. You have probably heard people say they lose their strength as they grow older. That is because as we age, we naturally lose muscle mass. New evidence shows that eight to 12 weeks of progressive weight training can significantly increase muscle strength in women, even as they progress well into their 90s.

Exercise and Cardiovascular Health

When it comes to keeping your heart healthy, exercise is key. Just like the other muscles in your body, your heart becomes stronger and more efficient when it is exercised regularly. This does not mean that you have to engage in overly vigorous workouts.

A seven-year study conducted at the University of Minnesota showed that women who did moderate exercise like raking leaves, bowling, or playing golf once a week were 24% less likely to die prematurely from cardiovascular illness than women who did not exercise.

Women who participated in vigorous exercise, like running or swimming, more than four times a week had a 43% lower risk of premature death.

Not only does exercise strengthen the heart muscle, it also lowers LDL (bad) cholesterol and increases HDL (good) cholesterol. Finnish researchers found that the favorable cholesterol balance associated with exercise may reduce the risk of arteriosclerosis, or hardening of the arteries.

Another cardiovascular benefit of exercise is reduced blood pressure. A study at Duke University Medical Center in Durham, North Carolina, showed that overweight people could reduce their blood pressure to a normal level by combining exercise with weight loss.

Building Brain Power

Flexing your muscles doesn't benefit just the body; it benefits the brain as well. Researchers from Case Western Reserve University Medical School in Cleveland, Ohio, found that people who were less physically and mentally active were three times more likely to get Alzheimer's disease as they aged.

Researchers believe that when you exercise, your heart pumps more blood to your brain, thereby supplying oxygen and essential nutrients that prevent cognitive decline and improve mental clarity. In fact, a fit person can process up to twice as much oxygen as an unfit one.

Build a Habit

Unfortunately, many women in their 40s and 50s forgo much-needed physical activity for other responsibilities that involve career and care-giving. In a recent study published in *Health Psychology*, researchers at the Stanford Center for Research in Disease Prevention studied the exercise habits of 3,000 women. They found that only 9% of study participants engaged in any type of regular physical activity.

The good news is that making exercise a part of your life may be easier than you think. Two studies that appeared in the *Journal of the American Medical Association* show that lifestyle exercise, or activities you perform as part of everyday living, can be just as beneficial as structured exercise you might do at a health club. In one study, researchers at the Cooper Institute for Aerobics Research in Dallas divided subjects into two groups. One group performed 30 minutes a day of lifestyle activities like walking, climbing stairs, vacuuming, and leaf raking. The other group did structured workouts on treadmills and stair climbers five times a week for 20 to 60 minutes. At the end of two years both groups showed similar improvements in cardiovascular health and body-fat percentage. Within one year of the study, the lifestyle group had regained less weight than the structured group.

Exercise and Menopause

For many women the years leading up to and even including menopause are an ideal time to make positive lifestyle changes. Increasing your physical activity may help control a number of symptoms specifically associated with menopause, including fatigue, headache, hot flashes, and anxiety, plus changes in skin, hair, muscle tone, bone health, and even memory. It has been proven that exercise, good nutrition, and—if recommended by your doctor—hormone therapy, can help keep menopause symptoms at bay. Exercise may even make you feel better than you did before menopause!

Here is some specific clinical evidence about exercise and your health for the menopausal years.

Hot Flashes

The symptom most often associated with menopause is hot flashes. Physical activity has been proven to taper this annoying symptom. One study of more than 1,600 women found that sedentary women were twice as likely to have hot flashes as women who exercised. Another study found women experienced fewer hot flashes directly after a 45-minute aerobic workout.

Psychological Benefits

Sleep deprivation may be a source of depression during menopause, since estrogen deficiency can impair sleep. A moderate amount of physical activity can help you sleep better at night. What's more, physical activity can greatly reduce anxiety and stress brought on by menopause. Researchers at the University of Georgia found that women in a study felt less stressed after exercising on a stationary bike for 40 minutes.

If even the idea of aerobic exercise is beginning to make you anxious, you can relax. In another study, researchers at the University of Texas in Houston found that leisurely exercise, like gardening or walking the dog, is an even better way to combat stress and anxiety than aerobic fitness.

Getting Started

We all know someone who made that New Year's resolution to begin exercising and ran out and bought a lot of expensive equipment, only to quit a few months later. The good news is that embarking on an exercise program doesn't have to be drudgery. Even small doses of gentle physical activity can boost your health and your mood. You can get the exercise you need by doing something you already enjoy, such as hiking, swimming, playing racquetball, or a combination of activities. Chances are, if you have fun exercising, you'll stick with it.

I always tell my patients they will never "find" the time for wellness. You must grab it before anything else fills the schedule, even if you just start out with only a single minute. Begin with this minute and increase the time as your health becomes your greater priority.

Check with Your Doctor

Before you start exercising, be sure to check with your doctor to make sure you have no medical problems that pose a risk. Conditions such as coronary heart disease, arthritis, and diabetes may require specific types of exercise or limits on your levels of exertion. Your doctor can help determine which activities are best for you and how much exercise your body can handle.

Here are six tests your doctor should perform as part of your physical examination, along with some guidelines on how to interpret the results:

1. Blood pressure test: This painless test is essential for detecting high blood pressure, which can increase your risk of heart attack, stroke, heart failure, and kidney damage. Systolic pressure (the top number) indicates pressure inside your arteries during the maximum pulse of each heartbeat. Diastolic pressure (the bottom number) shows the pressure inside the blood vessels as the heart is at rest. The pulsation, or pulse, can be felt in several areas of the body and signifies the ebb and flow of the heart in action.

   Results: Your blood pressure should not exceed 140/90. Studies are now showing that a much lower number, like 120/70 or below, is preferable for maximum health.

2. Lipid profile: This simple fasting blood test measures your total cholesterol, LDL (low-density lipoprotein) cholesterol, HDL (high-density lipoprotein) cholesterol, and triglycerides (fats). High total and LDL cholesterol levels can raise the risk of fatty deposits within your arteries, increasing your risk of heart attack and stroke. Exercise will decrease both total and LDL cholesterol safely. HDL cholesterol prevents and eliminates deposits. A high level of HDL is good.

   Results: Your total cholesterol should be below 200, or even lower for more protection. Your LDL cholesterol should be under 130, and your HDL cholesterol should be above 45—the higher the better.

3. Electrocardiogram (EKG): This painless test is used to detect abnormal rhythms, enlargement of the heart muscle, or other possible injury to the heart muscle. It only takes a few minutes and is usually done in the doctor's office. The nurse, technician, or physician will attach electrodes to your body while you are

lying down. These measure the electrical impulses generated by your heart.

Results: By reading your EKG your doctor will be able to determine if there are any apparent contraindications to a safe and effective exercise routine.

4. Stress test: This test shows how well your heart handles work. It also helps your physician determine the kind of exercise that's best for you and what level of intensity you can safely achieve.

You will be asked to exercise, usually by walking on a treadmill, while the doctor or a technician monitors your continuous EKG, blood pressure, and pulse response. The exercise stress test begins at a moderate walk. The treadmill increases in speed and incline as the test progresses. If you are very well conditioned you will begin to run, slowly at first and then faster until the physician asks you to stop. As you become more conditioned, you will be able to continue on the treadmill for longer periods of time before fatigue sets in. Any chest pain, shortness of breath, nausea, or light-headedness signifies a potential problem and should be noted immediately during the test.

Your primary health care provider may not have a treadmill available in the office and may need to send you to a specialist, like a cardiologist, for the test. Be wary of HMO and managed care plans or doctors who say that the test is not indicated. True, the tests are not cheap; they take time, and they require the expertise of a doctor trained in knowing what to look for during and after the test. But this is one of the best tests you can take to assure you that you can begin an exercise program without the fear of injuring your heart.

Results: A negative result on the exercise stress test is good. It means that nothing of concern happened to your heart under the period of stressful exercise you just completed. A positive exercise stress test means that there were unexpected changes seen on the heart monitor, including changes in your blood pressure or pulse.

5. Bone density measurement: This test is known as a DEXA (dual energy X-ray absorptiometry) and consists of an X-ray scan of your lower back and hip region, or another part of your skeleton, to detect loss of bone mass. This tests takes about 10 minutes and exposes you to less radiation than the average chest X-ray.

A different method tests bone density in the heel of your foot using ultrasound. This painless test entails inserting your foot into a box called the Sahara Clinical Bone Sonometer for 10 seconds while ultrasound measures bone density. This test is cheaper and faster than the DEXA, but it is not yet known how well it predicts the potential of hip and spine fractures, two areas measured directly by the X-ray method.

Bone density tests produce a "T-score" –for your bones, rating them from –1 or better (the density of a healthy 35-year-old) to –2.5, which indicates risk for osteoporosis. A score lower than –2.5 will usually result in a diagnosis of osteoporosis.

Your physician may recommend this test before you begin a fitness regime, since low bone density can lead to fractures, especially during physical activity.

Not all women are at equal risk for developing osteoporosis. Women who weigh less than 154 pounds, or who don't take supplemental estrogen, should be screened for osteoporosis beginning at the age of 60, according to a September 2002 statement by the U.S. Preventive Task Force. The task force also recommended that all women screened regularly beginning at age 65.

In addition, The National Osteoporosis Foundation recommends bone density testing if you have one or more risk factors for the disease:

- Low body weight
- Low calcium intake
- Poor health
- Family history of osteoporosis
- Previous fracture
- Smoker
- Alcohol abuser
- Frequent user of certain medications including steroids and thyroid hormones
- Caucasian or Asian descent

Approximately 50% of women over the age of 50 have signs of osteoporosis, so it is good to catch this disease early. By following a physician-prescribed program of exercise, calcium supplementation, and possibly additional medication, osteoporosis can be slowed, stopped, or even reversed.

6. Body mass index (BMI): Your BMI indicates your ratio of body fat to lean mass. BMI is used to predict your risk of heart disease, stroke, diabetes, and certain cancers. Use your height and weight to locate your BMI on tables. You can track your BMI to give yourself an objective measure of your improvement as you progress with your exercise program.

Results: If your BMI is 25 to 29.9, you are considered overweight. If your BMI is 30 and above, you are considered obese. A BMI lower than 18.5 indicates that you are underweight.

Getting Started

The doctor has cleared you; you are ready to jump right in and begin exercising in earnest. Not so fast! You may be skipping one of the most important aspects of your workout: the warm-up. Begin each exercise session by walking or jogging in place and then gently stretching your muscles. A 10- to 15-minute warm-up will loosen your muscles and reduce your risk of muscle injury or soreness. You will also find that flexibility exercises will increase the range of motion in your joints, keep your muscles limber, make you feel more relaxed, and improve your posture. Stretch slowly, exhaling as you stretch the muscle and inhaling as you relax. Hold each position for 10 to 30 seconds to the point of mild discomfort, but stop if you feel pain. Don't bounce while stretching, as this will only strain your muscles.

Time for Aerobics

Once you have limbered up your muscles, you are ready to start exercising.

If you want an exercise regime that will provide the greatest benefits to your heart and give you the most help in managing your weight, you will need to choose an aerobic activity such as brisk walking, jogging, or jumping rope.

You can determine how hard you are working out by measuring your heart rate as soon as you stop exercising. Simply count your pulse for 10 seconds (place two fingers against the pulse at either your wrist or the side

Body Mass Index Table

	NORMAL						OVERWEIGHT										OBESE
BMI	19	20	21	22	23	24	25	26	27	28	29	30	31	32	33	34	35
Height (inches)																Body Weight	
58	91	96	100	105	110	115	119	124	129	134	138	143	148	153	158	162	167
59	94	99	104	109	114	119	124	128	133	138	143	148	153	158	163	168	173
60	97	102	107	112	118	123	128	133	138	143	148	153	158	163	168	174	179
61	100	106	111	116	122	127	132	137	143	148	153	158	164	169	174	180	185
62	104	109	115	120	126	131	136	142	147	153	158	164	169	175	180	186	191
63	107	113	118	124	130	135	141	146	152	158	163	169	175	180	186	191	197
64	110	116	122	128	134	140	145	151	157	163	169	174	180	186	192	197	204
65	114	120	126	132	138	144	150	156	162	168	174	180	186	192	198	204	210
66	118	124	130	136	142	148	155	161	167	173	179	186	192	198	204	210	216
67	121	127	134	140	146	153	159	166	172	178	185	191	198	204	211	217	223
68	125	131	138	144	151	158	164	171	177	184	190	197	203	210	216	223	230
69	128	135	142	149	155	162	169	176	182	189	196	203	209	216	223	230	236
70	132	139	146	153	160	167	174	181	188	195	202	209	216	222	229	236	243
71	136	143	150	157	165	172	179	186	193	200	208	215	222	229	236	243	250
72	140	147	154	162	169	177	184	191	199	206	213	221	228	235	242	250	258
73	144	151	159	166	174	182	189	197	204	212	219	227	235	242	250	257	265
74	148	155	163	171	179	186	194	202	210	218	225	233	241	249	256	264	272
75	152	160	168	176	184	192	200	208	216	224	232	240	248	256	264	272	279
76	156	164	172	180	189	197	205	213	221	230	238	246	254	263	271	279	287

Source: Adapted from *Clinical Guidelines on the Identification, Evaluation, and Treatment of Overweight and Obesity in Adults: The Evidence Report.*

of your neck), and then multiply that number by six to determine your heart rate for one minute. The American Heart Association (AHA) recommends that you stay within 50–75% of your maximum heart rate. This range is called your target heart rate.

The following chart from the National Heart, Lung, and Blood Institute (NHLBI) can help you find your estimated target heart rate zones. Your maximum heart rate is about 220 minus your age.

If you don't like taking your pulse while you exercise, another way to maintain the appropriate level of effort is to use a conversational pace. If you can walk and have a conversation at the same time, you are not work-

				EXTREME OBESITY														
36	37	38	39	40	41	42	43	44	45	46	47	48	49	50	51	52	53	54
(pounds)																		
172	177	181	186	191	196	201	205	210	215	220	224	229	234	239	244	248	253	258
178	183	188	193	198	203	208	212	217	222	227	232	237	242	247	252	257	262	267
184	189	194	198	204	209	215	220	225	230	235	240	245	250	255	261	266	271	276
190	195	201	206	211	217	222	227	232	238	243	248	254	259	264	269	275	280	285
196	202	207	213	218	224	229	235	240	246	251	256	262	267	273	278	284	289	295
203	208	214	220	225	231	237	242	248	254	259	265	270	278	282	287	293	299	304
209	215	221	227	232	238	244	250	256	262	267	273	279	285	291	296	302	308	314
216	222	228	234	240	246	252	258	264	270	276	282	288	294	300	306	312	318	324
223	229	235	241	247	253	260	266	272	278	284	291	297	303	309	315	322	328	334
230	236	242	249	255	261	268	274	280	287	293	299	306	312	319	325	331	338	344
236	243	249	256	262	269	276	282	289	295	302	308	315	322	328	335	341	348	354
243	250	257	263	270	277	284	291	297	304	311	318	324	331	338	345	351	358	365
250	257	264	271	278	285	292	299	306	313	320	327	334	341	348	355	362	369	376
257	265	272	279	286	293	301	308	315	322	329	338	343	351	358	365	372	379	386
265	272	279	287	294	302	309	316	324	331	338	346	353	361	368	375	383	390	397
272	280	288	295	302	310	318	325	333	340	348	355	363	371	378	386	393	401	408
280	287	295	303	311	319	326	334	342	350	358	365	373	381	389	396	404	412	420
287	295	303	311	319	327	335	343	351	359	367	375	383	391	399	407	415	423	431
295	304	312	320	328	336	344	353	361	369	377	385	394	402	410	418	426	435	443

ing too hard. On the other hand, if you can sing while exercising, you are probably not exerting yourself enough, according to the AHA. If you have to stop to catch your breath, then chances are you are overdoing it.

As you near the end of your workout, you should gradually decrease your intensity. Keep moving for five to 10 minutes to cool down your muscles, then stretch them. This cool-down period will help prevent muscle soreness later on.

Strength Training

In addition to aerobic exercise, you should add strength or weight training to your routine. Doing calisthenics or using free weights or machines for about 20 minutes, two to three times a week, is recommended to build muscle and bone strength. Strength training also increases your muscle mass, which helps your body burn calories while at rest. As your muscle mass increases, you'll find it will be easier to maintain a healthy body weight.

If you choose to lift weights, begin with a weight that you can comfortably lift and progress slowly. Do one set of resistance exercises (eight to 12 repetitions), targeting each major muscle group of the upper and lower body.

Lift the weight to a count of two, and lower it to a count of four. Breathe by exhaling on the lift and inhaling on the release.

Be sure to consult with a certified fitness instructor to develop a program that meets your individual needs. It is also important to learn the proper technique and make sure you understand all safety guidelines so that you do not injure yourself.

How Much Is Enough?

The American College of Sports Medicine recommends 20 to 60 continuous or accumulated minutes of aerobic exercise three to five days per week; strength training, using free weights or machines, two to three days per week; and flexibility training two to three days per week. But this is your goal, not necessarily your starting point. Begin with only as much as you think you will be able to handle, and then add additional time in small increments.

Remember, the key to a successful exercise program is consistency, not how much you do. Overdoing it in the beginning may cause strains or injuries, or it might make you want to quit exercising altogether!

It's All in the Timing

Many women will tell you they use their exercise to wake up in the morning and start the day off right. Others prefer to take a time out during their

TABLE 6.1
Target Heart Rates

AGE (YEARS)	TARGET HEART RATE ZONE (50–75% OF MAXIMUM) BEATS PER MINUTE	AVERAGE MAXIMUM HEART RATE BEATS PER MINUTE
20	100–150	200
25	98–146	195
30	95–142	190
35	93–138	185
40	90–135	180
45	88–131	175
50	85–127	170
55	83–123	165
60	80–120	160
65	78–116	155
70	75–113	150

Credit: National Heart, Lung, and Blood Institute

noon hour to separate their morning from the afternoon. Some use the time after work to unwind from a day of toil. Still others take to the streets, gym, or treadmill in the evening to relax themselves before a shower and restful slumber. Whatever fits your fancy, getting your body in motion may be just the potion you have been seeking to help cure your stress woes.

Sticking with It

Exercise may keep our bodies looking young and healthy, but only if we do it regularly. In order to make exercise a habit, you need to make it a part of your lifestyle. Here's how:

- **Don't stop to question.** People who exercise regularly liken the activity to brushing their teeth or taking a shower. It is simply something they must do every day. Do you ever ask yourself whether you need to brush your teeth in the morning? Of course not. Treat exercise the same way.

- **Understand your motives.** Ask yourself why you want to exercise. Most women reading this book are thinking of exercising to overcome stress. But there are other reasons to exercise. Is it to look and feel younger? Wear clothes you can't fit into? Avoid your family history of heart disease? Once you know why you want to exercise, you'll be more likely to get up and get moving.
- **Keep a diary.** You may expect instant results, but chances are it will take weeks to months before you see an improvement. By tracking your progress—minutes of aerobic activity, number of miles walked, how much weight you lifted—you can watch your result unfold each day!
- **Expect setbacks.** When you first begin an exercise routine, you may find there are days when you just don't feel like continuing. Try a new activity or take a break. It may be that you were doing too much too soon.
- **Find activities you enjoy.** In order to keep it up, you've got to love—or at least enjoy—doing it. So if you find something you enjoy doing, chances are better that you will stay motivated.
- **Exercise with a friend.** No one wants to get up at the break of dawn to go jogging. But if you have a buddy, it will be much more fun.
- **Don't overdo it.** If you do too much too soon, you may get discouraged, sore, injured, or just plain bored. Think little steps . . . but keep taking steps. Don't stop.
- **Don't compare yourself to anyone else.** Just do the best you can and pat yourself on the back for getting out there and exercising.
- **Reward yourself.** You may find that increased fitness and a more youthful body are rewards enough. Still, a new pair of sneakers or a new jogging outfit might make your next workout a little easier.

A Final Word to the Stressed

One of the best weapons against overwhelming and out-of-control stress is to unwind the built-up tension with active movement. Get up, get moving, and watch the results unfold. You will see how a little investment yields great returns.

Liza's Progress

I want to end this chapter by letting you know how things worked out with Liza. Although she has not yet reached her weight loss goal as of this writing, she has lost 79 pounds and counting. Her three-month blood glucose level is now in the acceptable range (<200 mg/dl), down from well over 300 mg/dl when she first came in. Her cholesterol, previously over 250, is now 160 (<200 is considered normal), and her triglycerides are 69, where they were once nearly 300 (<150 is considered normal). Her fasting insulin is normal at 9.9 Uu/ml. The best part is that Liza feels better than she has in many years. She feels in control, and her stress level has decreased to a moderate and acceptable level.

Maybe you are not exactly like Liza. You may not be overweight or have her health problems. But she is an inspiring example for this chapter because if she could be successful, with all the hurdles she had to overcome, you can, too!

CHAPTER TEN

Step 6: Sensible Eating

Eating is one of the activities over which we should have total control, yet many women feel that food is controlling them. When life gets stressful or hectic, they reach for a candy bar or some other treat, and they continue to eat even after they have satisfied their hunger.

That kind of eating, called unconscious eating, is more about eating to satisfy emotional needs and to offset the effects of poor food and lifestyle choices than about satisfying hunger. For many it is almost unavoidable.

We all know people who engage in unconscious eating—perhaps even ourselves—but I will provide an example from my own practice.

A patient I will call Angela came in complaining of sudden weight gain. She had recently begun a new job, she said, and suddenly started gaining weight. She wondered if she had a metabolic disease. Could she have diabetes?

I gave her a blood sugar test, which came back normal. So did her thyroid tests. In addition, I asked her to keep a diary of everything she ate during the day for seven days, and then to bring in the food log so we could assess it together.

On her next visit she seemed embarrassed. Looking at the food log, I could see why. A colleague at Angela's new job kept a dish stocked with sweets. Without even noticing, Angela had been eating candy all day long. She didn't become aware of her behavior until she started keeping her food log.

Why we eat when we are not hungry is not completely clear. Some researchers feel that it is a nervous habit, like biting fingernails. People put food in their mouths to get rid of nervous energy. Other researchers think that stress causes a rapid depletion of blood sugar and that we eat fast food and other sugary, fattening snacks to raise those levels as quickly as possible.

Fluctuations in hormones can also cause a rise in unconscious eating. Low levels of serotonin (a neurotransmitter that, among other things, helps keep us from becoming depressed) can push people, especially women, to crave chocolate, which has an immediate calming effect. Others of us eat socially, to celebrate good times and to quench the despair of bad times. Many times food is used as a pacifier to fill in the boredom or alleviate the pressures caused by excessive stress.

We also have many opportunities for unconscious eating. Food gets center stage at many activities, and often hosts put little conscious effort into making healthy menu selections. Sometimes we do not even enjoy unhealthy treats as we are eating them.

The sad thing about eating when we are not hungry is that it leads to a vicious cycle that creates weight gain, which leads to even more emotional and physical stress, which can lead to more self-calming unconscious eating.

Conscious eating, on the other hand, involves learning to think about what you are eating, and why. Our nutritional choices influence literally every function in our bodies. What we eat and when we eat it also has a direct impact on how we manage the stress in our lives.

Is Your Attitude Toward Food Out of Control?

Take this test to see whether you control food, or food controls you.

1. Do you cope with stress by eating when you are not hungry?
2. Do you have difficulty differentiating true hunger from the desire to eat for comfort, out of boredom, or when you are anxious?
3. Do you see yourself as being overweight, even when others assure you that you're not?
4. Have you lost and regained the same pounds (plus a few extra) multiple times?
5. Do you weigh yourself once a day (or more)?
6. Do you feel like a failure if you have gained weight, even if you have gained only one or two pounds?

7. When you weigh yourself, do you feel as though weight lost is validation of your self-worth?

8. Do you skip meals to lose weight, but then find yourself overeating later in the day?

9. Do you try every diet you hear about, even if it goes against common sense—not to mention the basic rules of good nutrition or good health?

10. Do you find that you follow periods of strict dieting with periods of overeating?

11. Do you hide food for yourself or indulge in secret eating?

12. Do you plan what you will eat later in the day, even as you are eating an earlier meal?

13. Do you avoid certain situations because you fear the temptation to overeat will be too great?

14. Do you avoid going out in order to stay near food?

15. Does your closet contain clothing in a range of sizes to accommodate your fluctuating weight?

16. Do you lie about your weight?

If you answered yes to 6 or more of these questions, you need some help to become a more conscious eater and develop a positive body image.

In this chapter I am going to help you learn to accomplish those goals.

Body Weight and Self-Esteem

For many women, the best barometer of stress is body weight. The higher their level of stress, the more weight they gain. The heavier they become, the worse they feel about themselves, regardless of how intelligent, accomplished, loved, or otherwise successful they may be. Their weight and eating behavior become stressors in themselves.

The stress is exacerbated by the fact that women today hold themselves to an unrealistic image of beauty. Day in, day out, they are bombarded with media images showing them how they should look and dress. But those images are not true to life. Without their professional makeup, wardrobe, and flattering camera angles, most television and movie actresses would probably be unrecognizable in real life. The photographs of the models in those beautiful fashion magazines have probably been computer-enhanced to make the waists smaller, breasts "perkier," and complexions wrinkle and blemish free.

How Did We Get Here?

In the 1950s and 1960s magazines commonly carried advertisements for potions and supplements to increase body weight. And long before Twiggy walked her flat frame down the fashion runways of London, Marilyn Monroe set the standard of beauty in this country with her curves.

But the 1960s and 1970s were the years of great change for women. They began to question their traditional roles as housewives and mothers, and started entering the workplace, competing alongside men as their equals. They felt they should be able to take on all these new responsibilities without sacrificing any of their old ones—all the while continuing to look sexy and seductive for their men.

As women began trying to balance the competing demands of home, family, and career, they began experiencing new heights of stress. Many lived and worked great distances from family support networks, so they found themselves handling their responsibilities on their own. Although this was especially difficult for single mothers, many women began forgoing sleep, eating high-calorie fast food, and living on the run. The result? Weight gain. Coincidentally, those were also the key growth years for those segments of the food industry that focused on weight loss products such as diet soda, "skinny" bread, artificial sweeteners, and processed, prepackaged weight loss foods. A woman's weight became her central focus in finding the key to a successful modern life. She blamed her weight if she fell short of her goals for romance, professional advancement, fashion savvy, and social acceptance.

This situation continues today. Women worry. They worry about their ability to manage and achieve at work and to raise smart, self-sufficient children. They are anxious about themselves and the responsibilities of so-called sandwich generation women in caring for children and elderly relatives at the same time. They worry about saving enough money for retirement and for college. They see their responsibilities and obligations mounting and feel their ability to cope diminishing.

For many of these women eating is a refuge. The simple, soul-satisfying crunch of a stack of cookies or the succulent slurp of a milk shake is a quick, readily available way to nurture and comfort themselves.

The vast majority of these women would like to shed the extra pounds they have added, but they cannot break the vicious cycle of feeling stressed, eating, and feeling even more stressed.

Anxious Eating

Anxiety can foster an irresistible urge to eat. But eating does not cure anxiety, any more than thumb sucking, shopping, or nail biting does. It merely provides a temporary outlet.

Unfortunately, the bad feelings tend to return in force, especially if anxiety-induced overeating results in weight gain. For many women, weighing more than some arbitrary, idealized number is a badge of personal failure. It is an indication that they are weak, worthless, and lacking in self-control.

The Weight Loss Dilemma

Ironically, as women hold themselves to an increasingly stringent standard of thinness, Americans as a whole are becoming larger and larger. While the women in the Miss America Pageant have shown a 7% percent decrease in weight over the past 15 years, the average American woman has had an increase of 3–5% in body weight. Even the height/weight charts have changed, increasing the minimums and extending the maximum to 10–12 pounds beyond their upper limits of 20 years ago.

Recent studies conducted by the National Institutes of Health show that between 1998 and 1999 the prevalence of obesity in the United States climbed from 17.9 to 18.9% for all Americans. Obesity has increased among men and women of all races and socioeconomic groups, but it is a particular problem for women. An estimated 50% of American women are overweight.

Given those figures, it is no surprise that at any given time some 200 million Americans are trying to lose weight. Women have a corner on this particular market. By the time they have reached age 13, 80% of young girls report having already dieted, as compared with 10% of boys the same age.

Unfortunately, of all men and women who manage to shed pounds, 90–98% gain them back. That is why the business of weight loss is so lucrative. Americans are estimated to spend between $35 and $50 million a year on weight loss products.

Weight Loss for Your Health

Medical professionals weigh in on the side of keeping weight down. The predominant medical opinion is that excess body weight is a leading cause of disease. Research links excess body weight to a higher incidence of certain types of cancer, diabetes, stroke, high blood pressure, and osteoarthritis, as well as cardiovascular disease.

However, most research in this area is based on studies of people who already weigh more than the charts say they should. Little objective study has been conducted involving thin people who have become overweight and then develop these conditions and diseases. The question remains: Did they develop these diseases because they were overweight, or were they predisposed to developing these diseases and was being overweight an unrelated factor?

A related issue that deserves study is the potentially negative effect of dieting itself, as well as the effect of so-called yo-yo dieting (losing weight and then gaining it back again, over and over) on health and longevity. Preliminary studies conducted by the American Heart Association on yo-yo dieting have found that people whose weight fluctuates frequently through dieting have a much greater chance of developing heart disease than people whose weight is not subject to such fluctuations. More studies are needed on this important subject.

What Should You Believe?

Women are bombarded by a constant flow of information and misinformation about diet and exercise and how to keep their calorie and fat intake in check.

In the 1970s oat bran was touted as the panacea. Reported to absorb cholesterol like a sponge and whisk it safely away from the body's fat cells, grocery stores couldn't keep enough of the stuff on the shelves. Somehow, no one seemed to notice that some oat bran products also included palm oil, a saturated fat as unhealthy as lard and butter.

And what about eggs? The lowly egg was once damned as the dietary equivalent of Darth Vader—something no woman interested in her figure or her heart health would dream of eating. These days, in moderation, eggs are off the bad-guy list and are an accepted part of a balanced diet.

The bottom line is, don't sweat the headlines and try to resist the diet of the month. You should strive to eat a balanced diet, one that gains most of its calories (and bulk) from fruits and vegetables as well as whole grains. Protein, especially from animal sources, should appear on the plate in equal proportion to one serving of vegetables. Dairy products should be strictly low- or no-fat, and other fats and sweets should be kept to a minimum.

Oh No, Yo-Yo

To lose one pound of body weight, a woman must reduce her calorie intake by 3,500, increase calories burned by 3,500, or some combination of the two. That equation becomes more complicated as she ages. Due to hormonal changes, her body becomes less efficient at burning calories. At the same time, the distribution of her overall body fat changes, shifting to the abdomen, regardless of whether or not her body weight changes. In addition, as women age it grows increasingly likely that they will become less active, so they need to consume fewer calories to maintain the same weight.

The typical diet limits two things—carbohydrates and total calories. The result is short-term weight loss of a few pounds and then rapid weight gain, often to a level a pound or two above where the dieter started. How does this yo-yo effect happen?

It takes about three grams of water to store one gram of glycogen, a body's stored form of carbohydrate. High-protein, low-carbohydrate weight loss diets typically cause weight loss by eliminating glycogen and the water it takes to store it. They also tend to be low in calories, since food choices are so limited that the amount of food eaten automatically decreases. But losing glycogen reduces weight by eliminating some of the body's water, not its fat.

Meanwhile, diets that limit calories to less than about 1,200 a day fool the body into thinking it's starving. The body reacts by slowing its basal metabolic rate (BMR), the rate at which calories are burned while resting.

The longer you diet, the slower your BMR becomes. As BMR decreases, you lose weight more slowly. When you stop dieting and your calorie consumption returns to normal, renewed glycogen storage quickly adds lost water weight. In addition, your BMR remains low for a while, so you burn calories more slowly. These two factors may cause you to regain weight even more quickly after a diet, especially if you eat large quantities of formerly forbidden high-calorie, high-fat foods.

Why Fat Free Doesn't Work

Low-fat diets became the Holy Grail of dieting in the early 1980s, when the fact that a gram of fat provides nine calories (versus the four calories provided in a gram of carbohydrate or protein) started gaining attention.

Low-fat weight loss diets seemed to go hand in hand with healthy eating, since respected organizations such as the American Heart Association were advising us to consume no more than 30% of our day's total calories as fat calories. A study performed at the University of Colorado Health Sciences Center in 2000 seemed to reinforce the weight-loss benefits of a low-fat diet. There researches determined that 90% of excess fat calories consumed are converted to body fat compared to 70% of excess carbohydrates. It all seemed so obvious. There was no need to count calories as long as we were eating foods low in fat or completely devoid of it altogether. It would be good for our hearts and our waistlines.

Food manufacturers eager to claim a larger segment of the lucrative diet food marketplace jumped on the low-fat bandwagon. Suddenly, grocery store shelves were packed with low-fat and fat-free foods. Even foods that had never contained fat in the first place began to proclaim themselves fat-free tickets to the land of the slim.

But then two things became apparent. First, the bottom line about fat is that it makes food taste good. To compensate for the absence of taste in fat-free food, manufacturers increased the amount of sugar in many of these products. Sometimes, the net result was a fat-free food with considerably more calories overall than its fat-containing counterpart.

Then there was the issue of portion control. Researchers found that people ate much more of the fat-free foods than they would ever have eaten of the fat-containing versions. Larger portions meant extra calories—and weight gain.

The Problem with Diets

Many diets ignore the core issue of anxiety and its ability to lead some women to self-medicate with food. Instead they try to get people to switch from eating large quantities of high-calorie, fat-laden foods to unbalanced, large quantities of low-calorie, fat-free foods such as fruits and vegetables, or diet foods with little to no nutritional value. Or they shift the dieter into an unnatural world of program-based eating, such as all-protein or liquid diets. These are so alien to the way most of us normally eat that the people on these diets may as well be living on another planet. Eventually, though, the dieter returns to earth, feels deprived, and goes off the wagon, devouring large quantities of previously forbidden foods. The weight returns, often with a few additional pounds.

Healthy Eating

When my patients ask for healthy eating guidelines, I refer them to the Eating Plan for Healthy Americans that has been issued by the American Heart Association. It's based on years of medical research and is aimed at reducing the three major risk factors for heart disease and stroke—high blood cholesterol, high blood pressure, and excess body weight.

- Eat a variety of fruits and vegetables. Choose five or more servings per day.
- Eat a variety of grain products, including whole grains. Choose six or more servings per day.
- Include fat-free and low-fat milk products, fish, legumes (beans), skinless poultry, and lean meats.
- Limit your intake of cholesterol.
- Since not all fats are unhealthy, you need to pay attention not only to the *amount* of fat in your diet but also to the *type*. You should avoid (or limit) saturated fats (found in animal products such as red meat, whole milk, and butter) and trans fats, which are found in many margarines and prepared baked goods. Trans fats can increase your cardiovascular risk by raising the level of LDL (low-density lipoprotein) in your blood. It can be hard to tell if a prepared food contains trans fat since manufacturers are not required to list it on the label. However, you can tell if a food contains trans fat by looking for the words "hydrogenated fats" in the ingredient list.
- Your diet should include some heart-healthy omega-3 fats, which are found in foods like olive and canola oils, fatty fish such as

salmon and sardines, walnuts, flaxseeds, and flaxseed oil. These fats can *enhance* your health by helping to reduce your triglyceride levels and otherwise reducing your risk of cardiovascular disease.

- Balance the number of calories you eat with the number you use each day. (To find that number, multiply the number of pounds you weigh now by 15. This represents the average number of calories used in one day if you're moderately active. If you get very little exercise, multiply your weight by 13 instead of 15, as less active people burn fewer calories than more active individuals.)

- Maintain a level of physical activity that keeps you fit and matches the number of calories you eat. Walk or do other activities for at least 30 minutes on most days. To lose weight, do enough activity to use up more calories than you eat every day.

- Limit your intake of foods high in calories or low in nutrition, including foods like soft drinks and candy that have a lot of sugars.

- Eat less than six grams of salt (sodium chloride) per day (2,400 milligrams of sodium).

- Have no more than one alcoholic drink per day if you're a woman and no more than two if you're a man. "One drink" means that it contains no more than ½ ounce of pure alcohol. Examples: 12 oz. of beer, 4 oz. of wine, 1½ oz. of 80-proof spirits, or 1 oz. of 100-proof spirits.

Following this eating plan will help you achieve and maintain a healthy eating pattern. The benefits include a healthy body weight, a desirable blood cholesterol level, and a normal blood pressure. Not every meal has to meet all the guidelines. It's important to apply the guidelines to your eating pattern over at least several days. These guidelines may do more than improve your heart health. They may reduce your risk for other chronic health problems, including type 2 diabetes, osteoporosis (bone loss), and some forms of cancer.

A Fresh Viewpoint

What if you set aside all your preconceptions about your body and how much you ought to weigh? What if you took a fresh look at the process of managing your anxiety in a way that didn't involve numbing or nurturing yourself with food?

My proposed alternative would not ask you to avoid your inner hunger but to learn to manage it in new ways. It would mean putting aside your feelings that food and your body are malevolent forces working against you. Instead, you would learn to recognize them as symptoms about the ways you are living your life.

The following are suggestions for managing your weight, fostering a different view of your body, and initiating a lifelong process of living with the body you have. By creating an environment that is not so much based on denying yourself food as on finding new, healthier ways to live, you may discover important tools for coping with stress and fostering a life that nurtures you without resorting to unhealthy eating habits.

1. Tension of the Opposites

In her book *Addiction to Perfection,* Jungian analyst Marion Woodman speaks from personal experience about the ways that food can dominate the lives of those who use it to ease stress or to nurture themselves. She writes, "Overeating creates a concrete base with which the ego . . . is identified . . . the loss of body weight releases genuine anxiety and grief. . . ." It is one way to understand the all-too-frequent syndrome of yo-yo dieting that causes women to lose weight but be unable to maintain that weight loss.

Woodman, who had an eating disorder as a young woman, sees coming to terms with eating unrelated to hunger as an opportunity for spiritual exploration. Coining the phrase "holding the tension of the opposites," she asserts that eating when not hungry actually displaces deeper emotional needs and that actively engaging this emotional tension is an opportunity for self-discovery. She recommends using a journal to record dream images and "dialogue" with the waking and dreaming aspects of the self that lead to overeating.

2. Biblically Speaking

For those with strong traditional religious beliefs, the weight loss program Weigh Down may be an effective tool for weight loss and stress management. Often hosted at a variety of churches, its acolytes use a series of specially designed classes incorporating videos, audiocassette tapes, workbooks, and Bible lessons designed to help attendees "be delivered from the slavery of overweight."

This program teaches people that "head hunger" (the urge to eat when the body is not calling for food) is not true physiological hunger but rather spiritual hunger. The focus is on helping members learn how to replace head hunger with faith, a healthful diet, and exercise, along with prayer, Bible study, and companionship.

3. Twelve Steps

Overeaters Anonymous (OA), a 12-step program that mirrors Alcoholics Anonymous (AA), takes a broader, if no less spiritual, view to managing body weight. The program offers members support in dealing with the physical and emotional symptoms of compulsive overeating. Members are encouraged to seek professional help for individual diet and nutrition plans and for any emotional or physical problems.

Not a diet club, OA uses the AA one-day-at-a-time philosophy and is based on abstinence from overeating. Members admit that they have been unable to control compulsive overeating in the past and they must abandon the idea that all one needs to be able to eat normally is a little willpower.

As with AA, members attend meetings regularly and speak extensively on a voluntary basis about their struggles to cope, as well as share their successes. While the hat may be passed to cover the cost of coffee or room rental, there is no set charge for meetings.

4. Acupuncture and Universal Energy

Acupuncture, which has been practiced for more than 2,500 years in China, is based on an ancient technique in which a skilled practitioner inserts hair-thin needles into specific points on the body to prevent or treat illness. Practitioners of acupuncture view health as a constantly changing flow of energy, or qi (pronounced chee). Imbalances in this natural flow of energy are thought to result in disease and also may contribute to the urge to overeat. The goal of acupuncture aims to restore health by improving the flow of qi.

Acupuncture used to sound like hocus-pocus to the Western medical establishment. In the past decade, however, researchers have studied the effects of acupuncture on such diseases as high blood pressure, diabetes, stroke, certain nervous diseases, and various forms of pain, and have found it to be a highly effective form of treatment.

I have seen acupuncture used by patients to lose weight. One of my patients, a woman I will call Laura, when she decided to lose weight went to an acupuncturist on the advice of a friend. The acupuncturist described her excess weight as the result of unbalanced qi. Although Laura never completely understood what that meant, the result of several acupuncture treatments was a 25-pound weight loss.

5. Group Techniques

Numerous weight loss support groups, such as Weight Watchers, TOPS, Jenny Craig, and others, can be useful tools in managing weight. Most of these groups recommend a basic menu plan that generally mimics the guidelines of the FDA's Food Guide Pyramid. (For more information on the Food Guide Pyramid and the FDA dietary guidelines for Americans, see the U.S. Department of Agriculture Food and Nutrition Information Center Web site: http://www.nal.usda.gov/fnic/index.html.) These groups emphasize low-fat eating, carefully measured portions, and physical activity. Some have weekly lectures or private meetings with leaders to equip members with information about weight management techniques and to build a sense of support. They may heavily market their own prepackaged meals and snacks to members.

The camaraderie of weekly meetings with like-minded dieters, along with the commitment to be weighed and have that weight recorded, is intended to perpetuate a commitment to permanent lifestyle change. However, commitment is the operative word. Eventually, members must take responsibility for following program guidelines even when they are no longer attending meetings.

6. Prescription Weight Loss Aids

The use of prescription medication for weight loss and maintenance is still controversial, especially in light of the withdrawal of Phen-Fen, a popular combination weight-loss medication that was linked to a fatal pulmonary condition in some users. Drug therapies can help some people who are seriously obese, but they still do not take the place of diet, exercise, patience, and perseverance. Weight loss medication should always be used under a physician's supervision.

The majority of medications on the market today—Fastin, Ionamin, Bontril, Adipex-P, Meridia, and Desoxyn—limit appetite because of their effects on the hypothalamus, a control center in the brain. The shortcoming of this approach is that once patients stop taking the medication, the likelihood of regaining lost weight is substantial if lifestyle, eating, and exercise changes are also abandoned.

Prozac, an antidepressant, is the best-known member of the chemical family of drugs called selective serotonin reuptake inhibitors (SSRIs). SSRIs are FDA-approved for treatment of depression, bulimia, and obsessive-compulsive disorder, but are not specifically approved for weight loss. However, since some patients have reported weight loss with Prozac, doctors may prescribe it for this use. When used as directed in a comprehensive, physician-supervised weight loss program that includes a low-fat diet and regular exercise, Prozac is reported to enhance weight loss by about an additional 10%. However, this weight loss may not be permanent, especially after the Prozac has been discontinued.

None of these medications is cheap. When they are prescribed for weight loss, it's unlikely that an insurance company will pick up the tab. In addition, each medication carries with it a host of side effects and risk factors that should be discussed with your physician before taking this approach to weight loss.

7. Over-the-Counter Weight Loss Enhancers

In the 1950s and 1960s stimulants such as amphetamines were routinely prescribed for weight loss. However, the side effects, including anxiety, insomnia, and heart palpitations, made them fall from favor.

Now we know that nonprescription stimulants, ranging from the caffeine in coffee to Chinese ephedra (also known as ma huang) contain the stimulants ephedrine and pseudoephedrine. Both ephedrine and caffeine increase the basal metabolic rate. They also seem to depress appetite. And caffeine has a mild antidepressant and diuretic effect. I don't recommend taking ephedra under any circumstances, because it has been known to cause high blood pressure, cardiac arrhythmias, stroke, and even death. Many people who attempt weight loss on their own fail approximately 98% of the time. Supervised programs or physician-assisted weight loss programs have a much better success rate.

8. Practice Prohibition

While it is true that research seems to indicate that a glass of red wine with dinner may help keep cholesterol levels in check, it's also a fact that alcohol is high in calories and contains little, if any, nutritive value.

If a woman's daily routine includes alcohol, she is consuming an extra 100–300 empty calories per drink. Alcohol contains seven calories per gram, almost as much as the nine calories contained in a gram of fat and significantly more than the four calories in a gram of carbohydrate or protein. Multiply that by two or three drinks a day, or 14–20+ drinks a week, and it doesn't take long to reach the 3,500 calories that make up a pound of weight. More important, if alcohol is being used to take the edge off stress, it may be time to reassess its use as a potential addiction.

9. Water, Water Everywhere

There are lots of good reasons to drink water. Water flushes the kidneys, minimizing the chances of developing kidney stones. It hydrates the tissues and makes it easier for food to be digested. It also helps make you feel full. However, the body's signals of its need for water may be ones that compulsive eaters misinterpret or have learned to ignore.

Some nutritionists believe that compulsive eaters may confuse the body's need for hydration with the signal to eat. The next time you get an urge to snack even though you are not truly hungry, drink an eight-ounce glass of ice water. You may find that you are satisfied without having consumed a single calorie.

10. Hot Stuff

Can hot, spicy food increase basal metabolic rate? Researchers at Oxford Polytechnic Institute in England compared the metabolic rates of people when they consumed a standardized diet and again when they ate the same diet with a teaspoon each of red-pepper sauce and mustard added to every meal. They found that the spices caused a significant increase in the subjects' basal metabolic rates.

There is another weight-loss benefit from eating spicy foods. Hot food stimulates thirst, which causes you to drink more liquids. If you fill up on water instead of food, you ingest fewer calories. This may help you to lose weight.

11. Fill 'Er Up

Psyllium is the seed of the plantain plant. It is commonly available in bulk at health food stores and is an ingredient in many natural laxatives. Rich in fiber and a jellylike substance called mucilage, when psyllium comes in contact with water, the mucilage absorbs the fluid and expands substantially. In the stomach, psyllium expansion can produce feelings of fullness.

In one Italian study, researchers gave a group of seriously obese women specially prepared low-fat meals. Some of the women also took a few teaspoons of psyllium and water before the meals. The women who took the psyllium lost more weight than the women who did not take it.

12. Herbal Options (Serotonin Sources)

Serotonin is the chemical in the brain responsible for the feeling of full-ness. By increasing your serotonin, you feel fuller sooner and eat less. This may be why the antidepressant Prozac produces weight loss in some individuals.

A key ingredient in serotonin is the amino acid tryptophan. Some years ago injuries caused by a contaminated batch of tryptophan spurred the FDA to ban sales of this amino acid. However, you can still increase serotonin intake by consuming herbs rich in tryptophan or serotonin, notably evening primrose oil and especially walnut oil. Walnuts are one of nature's richest sources of serotonin. They are also high in fat, so you'd think they'd be a no-no for people interested in weight control. But a study of more than 25,000 Seventh Day Adventists showed that those individuals who ate the most walnuts were the least obese. Seventh Day Adventists are vegetarians who eat a diet considerably lower in fat than the average American.

Try adding some walnuts to your diet for a few weeks. See if you notice any difference in how easy or difficult it is to control your weight.

13. Online

The information superhighway has emerged as a high-tech tool for weight loss and management. A Brown University study compared two groups of dieters: one used an assortment of weight loss sites on their own to guide them in dieting; the other had access to the same sites plus the support of e-mailed behavior modification therapy from weight loss experts. They also maintained a record of calories, fat grams, and exercise, and they had access to a bulletin board for social support. After 12 weeks the information-only group lost an average of three pounds; the other group, nine. Researchers agree that while information alone doesn't help people change behavior, the difference between the two groups' levels of success might have been the additional resources the Web sites provided (chat rooms, cooking ideas, fitness plans, and food logs).

Four examples of weight-control Web sites are dietwatch.com, ediets. com, efit.com, and thriveonline.com/weight/. But if you are thinking of bringing a Web component into your weight management program, be sure to check out the privacy policies and be leery of sites that require extensive personal information. Web dieters should look for sites carrying content by credible medical professionals and beware of those that tie weight loss to the purchase of supplements and products.

14. Set Incremental Goals

Start out by setting small, attainable goals for yourself, and give yourself plenty of time to succeed. You may need to lose 50 pounds in all, but don't think about that right now. Give yourself three months to lose that first five pounds, and reward yourself when you've reached that goal. Buy yourself some flowers or a new lipstick. Set yourself another small, attainable goal. By the time you have reached this second one, you may find that you have lost so much weight that some of your clothes are a little loose on you. Why not reward yourself by buying a new blouse or a pair of jeans? It may even be a size smaller than what you are used to wearing! If you missed the mark, that's fine, too. Take three months off to learn how to maintain whatever loss you achieved and appreciate the fact that you've made progress toward the goal. You can even treat yourself to a (nonfood) reward for making a good attempt. Then set another five-pound, three-month goal.

If you set small incremental goals and reward yourself each time you reach one you will keep feeling good about yourself, no matter how long it takes for you to lose all your weight. But if your only goal is your ultimate target you will find yourself getting frustrated along the way. The more frustrated you get, the more difficult it will be to stick to your eating plan.

Rewarding yourself for achieving small successes will make it easier for you to follow the next guideline.

15. Slow and Steady

Nobody likes to hear it, but it is true. The more slowly you lose weight, the more likely you are to keep it off. There are a number of reasons for this.

First, as I have already explained, the typical 1,200 calorie weight loss diet feels like starvation to your body, so it adapts, becoming more efficient. Metabolism slows and so does weight loss. Go through this process often enough and researchers believe metabolism permanently gears down. Losing weight more slowly is less likely to slow your metabolism.

Second, you are more likely to stick with minor adjustments in your lifestyle. Giving up or cutting back on just a few of your favorites is less likely to trigger the bingeing that can occur when starvation or strict denial rule your life.

There are a host of other reasons that slow weight loss is more desirable than a rapid reduction plan. Losing weight slowly decreases the likelihood of sagging skin that can come with a too rapid weight loss. There's also the time required for the mental adjustment. How many times have you lost 20 pounds but looked in the mirror and seen the same overweight body? Slow weight loss gives your eyes and your mind the chance to adjust to the changes in your body. Finally, gradual weight loss allows you to firmly establish workable weight maintenance strategies that you will be able to sustain.

16. Stem the Tide

Rather than launching into yet another weight loss plan, consider focusing on maintenance. Discover what it would take to hold your weight at exactly what you weigh today. You may be surprised to learn how much your weight naturally varies from one day to the next, without any active effort to increase or decrease it. At the end of six months, if you still feel the need to lose weight, apply what you've learned about eating and exercise during maintenance to your efforts to lose.

17. Yes, You Know This One: Exercise

It is a well-established fact that people who exercise lose weight more quickly and generally feel better than people who do not exercise. They lose weight because exercise burns calories and because the body tends to continue burning calories at a higher rate even after you've stopped exercising. They also feel better because exercise brings about the release of increased amounts of endorphins, which are naturally occurring brain chemicals that lighten your mood. Exercise also feels good as a result of the increased oxygen made available to the tissues when you raise your heart rate and breathe deeply.

I devoted an entire chapter to exercising for stress reduction earlier in this book. Here I will just tell you that exercise does not have to be a formal activity. Just do something. Park your car in the far corner of the office parking lot and walk to the office entrance. Take the steps instead of the elevator. Do leg lifts during the commercials on your favorite television shows. Play fetch with the dog. Use hand weights while waiting for the coffee to drip. At the very least, you'll improve the mobility of your joints, increase muscle flexibility, and build strong bones. All of these are beneficial for your long-term health.

And Then There's Staying There

Diet books are filled with good ideas for losing weight, but few give more than a nod to the subject of maintenance. It's no wonder. Dieters can become so obsessed with weight loss that by the time they near or reach their goal weight, they're so sick of the process—denial, food measuring, living on expensive and unsatisfying diet foods—that they fall off the wagon with a crash. In addition, when stress gets out of hand most dieters fall back into a familiar, comfortable pattern of eating to soothe themselves.

While it's true that 90% of people who lose weight regain it, those who are successful have several characteristics in common:

- They made specific lifestyle changes that help them cope with stress in a more constructive way.
- Their weight loss was slow. The rule of thumb was once that we should aim to lose no more than two pounds per week. These days, nutritionists say two pounds per month makes more sense.
- They exercised during and after the weight loss. This does not mean that they became Olympic weight lifters or marathon runners. They simply found an exercise activity that they enjoyed doing and they stuck with it. Then they made that activity a part of their postdiet lives.
- They forgave (and forgive) themselves for occasional transgressions. Breakfast out on a Saturday morning did not become an excuse for bingeing all weekend. It was just breakfast. By noon they were back to healthy eating and exercise as usual.
- They paid attention to portion sizes rather than to calories.
- They found ways to deal with their hot buttons that triggered overeating. Did alcohol lead to overeating? They skipped cocktail hour. Was a certain time of day difficult to handle? They scheduled a noneating activity for that time.

If you use the information in this chapter to gain control over what you eat and how you see yourself when you look in the mirror, you will have conquered some of life's major stressors.

CHAPTER ELEVEN

Step 7: Sound Sleep

Sleep is an essential ingredient for good health. During sleep the brain repairs itself from the day's activities, rejuvenating your mind and body, making you feel refreshed. Sleep allows the brain to repair itself. If you don't sleep or if your sleep is interrupted or too short, this repair process is undermined.

Unfortunately, many people do not get enough sleep. They have difficulty falling asleep, wake up several times during the night, or arise too early in the morning. This is too bad, since sleep deprivation affects your personality, your ability to function, and your well-being. It causes fatigue, irritability, reduced attention, lower concentration, and impaired memory. Insufficient sleep can also make you more susceptible to illness or injury.

The Relationship Between Sleep and Stress

Sleep is a major factor in The Stress Cure, as few things can relieve stress as effectively as a good night's sleep. Yet sleep is one of the most difficult things to come by when you are under stress. This is what I call the sleep paradox, and it is especially common in women.

One such woman was a patient I'll call Sarah. Sarah was exhausted when the alarm sounded at 6:00 A.M. She shook her husband awake. As soon as he opened his eyes, a sympathetic look crossed his face.

"Didn't sleep too well again, dear?" he asked. Sarah shook her head, frustrated. She had lain awake, tossing and turning, until about 2:00 A.M. Then she had fallen asleep for an hour or two but had been awake ever since. She could not bear to watch her husband lying next to her, snoring happily, any longer.

Her husband had run out of suggestions long ago. And Sarah no longer had any sleep ideas of her own. She had tried counting sheep, soft music, no music, an eye mask to block out light, and several over-the-counter sleep aids.

Nothing seemed to help.

When she was trying to fall asleep, Sarah could not keep thoughts from racing through her mind. The more she tried to relax, the harder it became. Her early-morning awakening became more frequent, and she was rarely able to put herself back to sleep. By the time she came to see me, Sarah had become so sleep deprived that she feared she would soon become unable to drive or go to work. On the average she was getting only one night per week of normal slumber.

Sarah's lack of sleep was increasing her level of stress. The less she slept, the more irritable she became. This irritability caused her to feel anger, guilt, rage, and sadness all at the same time. When she went to bed, these feelings became overwhelming and kept her from sleeping. She was caught in a vicious circle she felt powerless to escape.

In reality, the stress in Sarah's life was not causing her sleeplessness. It was the other way around. After giving Sarah a physical examination and asking about her lifestyle habits, I discovered that she was taking antihistamines and decongestant products for allergies—too many, actually—and they were keeping her awake. One product contained pseudoephedrine, a common over-the-counter substance designed to open up the nasal passages. Sarah may as well have been drinking caffeine before going to bed, as the two substances have similar effects. All in all, her medication was preventing her from achieving a deep and restful sleep. The result was an increase in the amount of stress she experienced from things that had never affected her to such an extent.

The solution to Sarah's stress problem was easy. I prescribed a different antihistamine that was more effective, without the stimulatory effect, at a lower dose. Then I had her follow the remainder of the six-step stress cure that you find in this book, all with good results.

Not all sleep problems can be solved so easily. Some sleep problems can be complex in nature and very difficult to solve. If, after reading this chapter, you feel that your sleep problems are too complex to be solved by this program, I recommend contacting a sleep center where experts in this new field of medicine may choose to have you sleep over in one of their facilities so they can determine the exact nature of your problem.

The purpose of this chapter is to provide a broad overview of the importance of sleep in your life. Then I will offer a variety of tips for solving your own slumber problems and making sure that you are getting the highest quality sleep possible.

Slumber Is Scarce for Many

According to William Dement, M.D., chairman of the Sleep Disorder Clinic at Stanford University School of Medicine, "A substantial number of Americans, perhaps the majority, are functionally handicapped by sleep deprivation on any given day." A recent sleep survey conducted by the National Sleep Foundation confirms this belief. The survey found that one-third of all adults in the United States get fewer than six and a half hours of sleep per night. Medical experts recommend that we sleep eight hours per night.

Women are especially prone to sleep disturbances. An astonishing three-fourths of women sleep fewer than eight hours each night during the week, and fewer than seven hours per weekend night! And insomnia affects women at every age. According to the National Sleep Foundation survey,

- 71% of premenopausal women report insomnia during their menstrual periods,
- 56% of menopausal women report frequent insomnia symptoms, and
- 79% of pregnant women report that their sleep is more disturbed during pregnancy than when they were not pregnant.

The Hormonal Effects of Sleep Deprivation

Sleep deprivation can increase stress hormones such as cortisol and adrenocorticotropin, causing you to feel tired and stressed after a night of little or poor-quality rest. A study conducted at the National Institutes of Health in Bethesda, Maryland, found that insomniacs had higher concentrations of stress hormones than other participants, both day and night. As we know, prolonged increases in cortisol lead to depleted DHEA levels and a decreased ability to cope with life's stresses and problems.

Women are especially affected by sleep deprivation as it relates to stress hormones. Researchers at the University of Washington, Seattle, found that women who had impaired sleep had higher levels of cortisol than their rested cohorts.

Sleep Deprivation and Mental Acuity

Normally, we usually pass through five phases of sleep. The five-phase cycle repeats itself at 90- to 110-minute intervals. REM (rapid eye movement) sleep, in which we spend about 20 to 25% of our total sleep time, is the fifth phase. In order to reap the full benefits of sleep, you must experience REM sleep. This is the most restorative sleep, and without it you will not feel refreshed upon waking.

Experts believe that sleep, especially deep sleep, enables our nervous system to function well. Without it, we lose our ability to concentrate, remember, or analyze. Severe sleep deprivation can lead to hallucinations and mood swings. Ironically, the intensive care unit (ICU) in the hospital is a prime example of where this can occur. ICU patients are frequently awakened many times during the night for blood tests, blood pressure checks, and various other treatments. After several days of being robbed of deep, restful sleep, ICU patients have been known to have psychotic episodes.

Some experts attribute the healing quality of sleep to the belief that it allows neurons an opportunity to regain energy and shed by-products of daily cellular activity. There has also been speculation that during deep sleep, cells manufacture more proteins, which are essential for cell growth and repair of damage from stress and ultraviolet rays.

Scientists believe that activity in the area of the brain that controls emotions and social interactions lessens during sleep and that deep sleep may help people be emotionally and socially adept when awake.

Sleep may also allow our brain to store a newly learned activity in its memory bank. Researchers at Johns Hopkins University found that after a person masters a physical skill, the brain needs up to six hours to transfer the memory of how to perform that skill from the learning center of the brain to its permanent storage banks. And sleep experts at Trent University in Peterborough, Ontario, found that sleep deprivation significantly affects learning. Students taught a complex logic game and then deprived of sleep the same night showed a 30% learning deficit when tested a week later compared to students not deprived of sleep.

While getting less sleep affords us more hours to accomplish our daily tasks, studies show that sleep deprivation actually makes us less able to function properly. In one national survey more than half of women reported that their sleep problems frequently interfered with their daily activities. Researchers say that fatigue brought on by lack of sleep compromises our performance and speed of accuracy.

Australian researchers found, for example, that sleep deprivation impairs cognitive and motor performance in the same manner as alcohol. So it is not surprising that drowsy drivers cause at least 100,000 car accidents each year, according to a report by the National Highway Traffic Safety Administration.

Studies have also confirmed that sleep deprivation affects memory and concentration. Sleep experts from the University of California, San Diego, School of Medicine revealed that people who were deprived of sleep for 35 hours scored lower on memory tests and experienced lower levels of concentration than did rested participants. German scientists found that sleep disturbances in astronauts significantly affected their cognitive and motor functioning. According to a survey by the National Sleep Foundation, more than six out of 10 respondents said their concentration was diminished when they were sleep deprived. And a study at the University of Pittsburgh Medical Center showed that losing sleep slows down thinking skills the next day.

Sleep Deprivation and Your Health

The effects of sleep deprivation on other bodily functions are just as alarming as the cognitive effects. In studies from five medical centers across the United States, researchers established that individuals with insomnia were also more likely to have poor health, including chest pain, arthritis, depression, and difficulty accomplishing daily tasks. Another breakthrough study revealed that even temporary loss of sleep can affect the body's ability to break down carbohydrates, interfere with the function of various hormones, and worsen the severity of age-related ailments such as diabetes and high blood pressure.

Some researchers believe sleep loss weakens the immune system, thus increasing vulnerability to disease. A recent study at the University of Tennessee found that sleep deprivation in rats led to suppression of the immune system, resulting in death. Whether or not the results of this study apply to humans is still to be determined.

The point of my presenting a summarized version of all of these studies is to give you a broad overview of why sleep is so important. But I don't think you need pages of medical studies to be convinced that you need a good night's sleep to feel your best during the day. It might not be the only factor that will make your waking hours pleasant and stress free, but it is certainly the foundation for stress-free living.

What Causes Insomnia?

At the beginning of this chapter, I described the stress paradox—the vicious cycle by which stress prevents sleep, one of the very best remedies for stress. But stress is not the only factor keeping us awake.

Technology
For some people the high-tech phenomenon of being instantly accessible robs us of sleep. When our cell phones, fax machines, and pagers ring morning, noon, and night, we feel compelled to respond.

Overscheduling
Insomnia may result from a compulsion to try to accomplish more in a 24-hour day than is realistic. In fact, a startling 45% percent of adults say they sleep less in order to accomplish more. Often there simply is not enough time to accomplish all the work, household chores, child care, and other responsibilities of daily life, so people whittle away at their sleeping time.

In the last two decades, for example, Americans have tacked on more than 150 hours to their work and commute times.

Ignoring Your Internal Clock
Our bodies are naturally programmed with circadian rhythms, which govern the various systems in our body, including the 24-hour sleep/wake cycle, body temperature, hormone secretion, blood pressure, and even urine production.

Each of these systems is regulated by an internal biological clock. Located in the brain, this clock is called the suprachiasmatic nucleus (SCN), and it is composed of 20,000 neurons. When it grows dark outside, signals from the SCN are transmitted to the pineal gland, which stimulates the production of melatonin, also known as the hormone of sleep. Melatonin is made and released only when the brain senses nighttime conditions. Your rising melatonin level causes you to feel drowsy.

Sometimes our lives require us to work out of sync with our internal clock, causing disturbances in our sleep patterns. We may be morning larks required to stay up late, or we may be night owls who have to get up at the crack of dawn. This disruption of our natural sleep/wake cycle may cause us to feel groggy or stressed during the day.

Psychological Factors
New evidence shows that 14% of people with insomnia also suffer from depression. Sleep disturbance is a key symptom of depression. There is also a strong link between insomnia and psychiatric conditions like schizophrenia, anxiety disorders, and manic-depression (or bipolar disorder). Studies show that 25–65% of bipolar patients with a manic episode experienced a sleep disruption prior to the episode.

Sleep Apnea
One of the most well researched sleep disorders is sleep apnea, a breathing disorder affecting an estimated 18 million Americans. There are three types of sleep apnea:

- Obstructive sleep apnea, a common problem, occurs when the muscles in the back of the throat relax to the point where they obstruct your breathing and cause loud snoring. This can happen repeatedly throughout the night.
- Central sleep apnea occurs when the brain forgets to signal to the breathing muscles that it is time to move. The lack of oxygen causes the brain to wake the sleeping person.
- Mixed sleep apnea, which is a combination of obstructive and central sleep apnea.

One of the major risk factors for sleep apnea is obesity. Excess fat can accumulate in the upper airway and tongue, serving to close off the airway. In some overweight people the upper airway is shaped differently, which may add to its ability to collapse. Other factors leading to sleep apnea are narrow nasal passages, small facial bones, or extremely soft tissues at the back of the throat.

Since sleep apnea causes continual waking, many sufferers experience irritability or depression during the day due to disrupted sleep patterns. Apnea reduces oxygen intake, so it can also lead to headaches, a loss of interest in sex, or reduced mental performance. Sleep apnea may also lead to cardiovascular disease.

Researchers at the University of Wisconsin School of Medicine in Madison found that sleep-disordered breathing may be a risk factor for hypertension and, consequently, heart disease. In rare cases sleep apnea can lead to sudden death caused by respiratory arrest.

The good news is that there are many treatments for sleep apnea. If the symptoms are mild, simply losing weight or sleeping on your back can help.

Dental appliances worn at night to reposition the tongue or jaw may also be useful. For obstructive apnea, a device known as a CPAP (continuous positive airway pressure) can help maintain airflow during the night.

Restless Legs Syndrome

Another sleep disorder, restless legs syndrome (RLS), is characterized by uncomfortable prickling or tingling sensations in the thighs or calves.

People with RLS often have the urge to move their legs for relief and may constantly move their legs throughout the night. RLS, which affects 12 million Americans, is sometimes associated with anemia, pregnancy, or diabetes.

Many people with RLS also suffer from periodic limb movement disorder (PLMD), causing repetitive jerking or twitching movements, usually in the lower limbs. Sleep experts believe PLMD is sometimes linked to kidney disease, diabetes, or anemia. Occurring every 20 to 40 seconds, these rapid movements can cause sufferers to awaken frequently throughout the night.

There are several medications used for PLMD and RLS, including dopaminergic or opioid drugs, anticonvulsants, benzodiazepines, and baclofen.

Gastroesophageal Reflux

Another common cause of insomnia is gastroesophageal reflux, commonly known as heartburn. This is a condition in which stomach acid backs up into the esophagus.

New research from the American Gastroenterological Association shows that nearly eight in 10 people with heartburn have symptoms during the night, causing them to lose sleep. Forty percent of participants reported that the sleep loss affected their ability to work the next day.

Sleep Terrors

One of the most frightening disorders is the onset of intense fear in the middle of the night, also known as night terrors. People with this disorder wake up suddenly, often screaming and kicking. Each episode lasts about 15 minutes and is usually not remembered the next morning.

REM Movement Disorder

Another condition that may disturb sleep is REM movement disorder. REM movement disorder also causes those affected by it to display violent physical behavior. Normally during REM sleep your body assumes a temporary state of paralysis, which ends when you wake up. However, in REM movement disorder, the paralysis does not occur. This allows the sleeper to act out dreams or nightmares. Unlike people with sleep terrors, people with REM movement disorder recall their dreams. Medications have proven to be effective in treating this disorder.

Snoring

One sleep disorder that sounds benign but may actually have serious implications is snoring, which affects more than a third of all adults. Not only could snoring indicate sleep apnea, it is also linked to high blood pressure. Sleep researchers at the Penn State College of Medicine in Hershey, Pennsylvania, found that people who snore are one and a half times more likely to have high blood pressure, which can lead to heart disease and stroke. Snorers with even mild sleep apnea were two and a half times more likely to have high blood pressure. The risk for those with moderate to severe sleep apnea was seven times greater than for persons with no sleep problems.

Sleep Tips from the Sandman

The following tips will help you improve the quantity and quality of your sleep, allowing you to feel refreshed and rejuvenated in the morning:

- Get moving. Try to fit 20 to 30 minutes of exercise into your schedule each day. Exercise improves sleep by reducing stress, raising your blood oxygen level, and pumping up your body temperature, which can make you feel ready for sleep.
  Researchers at the University of Washington found that people

who ran or walked 40 minutes three days a week enjoyed longer periods of deep sleep than those who did not exercise. However, avoid exercising right before you go to bed, since this might interfere with your sleep. Sleep scientists at the University of Arizona in Tucson found that men and women who walked in excess of six blocks each day experienced a third fewer sleep problems such as insomnia than people who walked less. But women in the study who exercised late in the evening had difficulty falling asleep.

- Massage your muscles. A weekly massage can help alleviate insomnia, especially in people who suffer from painful disorders such as fibromyalgia and arthritis. A short massage from a spouse or partner can relax tight shoulders and help release serotonin, a feel-good brain chemical that helps bring on sleep.

- To relieve anxiety after a stressful day, plan time for relaxation with yoga. Yoga can improve your breathing, soothe away stress, and relax your nervous system. Try to practice yoga at the same time every day and you will associate it with a good night's sleep.

- Skip the caffeine and alcohol. Any drink that contains caffeine, such as coffee, soft drinks, or nonherbal teas, serves as a stimulant. Surprisingly, so does alcohol. Even though a glass of wine before bed may help you get to sleep faster, it can shorten your total sleep time and aggravate conditions such as heartburn and sleep apnea.

- Establish a pattern. Go to sleep the same time each night and get up at the same time each morning. Try to maintain this schedule throughout the week. Sleeping late on weekends can throw off your internal clock and make it difficult to return to your sleep schedule during the week.

- If you suffer from restless legs syndrome, try rubbing your legs before going to bed, walking around, or taking a hot shower or bath. Should you find that you feel excessively tired during the day, see your doctor.

- If gastroesophageal reflux (heartburn) is a problem, eat dinner earlier in the evening and avoid eating spicy or greasy foods before going to bed. Try drinking a glass of milk before going to sleep.

- Don't worry. Easier said than done, I know. But when you hit the pillow, try to forget about solving all your problems. Experts suggest writing down your worries before dozing off and placing the list where you can find it the next morning. If you get into bed and find that you just cannot relax, don't just lie there. Try reading, watching television, or listening to music until you feel drowsy enough to sleep. Above all, don't worry about not being able to fall asleep. Worrying can make your insomnia worse.

• It is normal to feel groggy in the afternoon sometimes. A nap can help you catch up on much-needed sleep, and it is much more effective than dozing longer on weekends. For greatest benefits, you should take your nap at about the same time every day, either midafternoon or about eight hours after you wake. As refreshed and energized as you might feel after a nap, know that it is not a substitute for a full night's sleep. Don't nap for more than 30 minutes at a time or you will fall into a deep sleep and feel drowsy upon waking. If you have difficulty sleeping at night, a daytime nap might aggravate the problem. Some people can feel refreshed after just a 10–15 minute nap; any longer than this and they feel groggier than when they closed their eyes. Experiment and find the optimum time for you to take an afternoon siesta.

• Monitor medications. Some prescription medications are known to cause insomnia. The biggest culprits are blood pressure drugs, hormones for thyroid disease and birth control, bronchodilators, decongestants, antihistamines, weight loss prescriptions, some herbal preparations, and pain medications containing caffeine.

• See the light. Make sure you get regular exposure to outdoor sunlight, especially in the morning when you wake up. Sunlight is necessary to keep your internal clock on track.

• Keep it cool and quiet. Adjust the temperature in your bedroom so that you stay cool at night. Try using a fan, air purifier, or white-noise generator (like the static from a radio not tuned to a station) to soothe away disruptive noises. If your clock ticks loudly or has a bright face, place it on a dresser on the other side of the room. This will also prevent you from checking the time. And make sure your bed is large and comfortable.

• Try not to eat too late at night. Eating a large meal close to bedtime can keep you awake. If you are hungry before bedtime, try foods containing the sleep-inducing amino acid tryptophan, found in milk, turkey, bananas, honey, tuna, egg whites, beans, peanuts, and green leafy vegetables. Avoid eating foods containing tyramine—bacon, cheese, sugar, ham, or tomatoes—which stimulate the brain and keep you awake.

- See your doctor. Much is known about sleep disorders, and your primary care physician can either help you or refer you to a sleep specialist. These days, most sleep disorders can be managed effectively once they are diagnosed.

    Don't wait for your doctor to ask about your sleep; take the initiative in talking about your sleep problems. Many doctors simply will not ask.
- Prescription medications. When all else fails, if you have tried various approaches to combating insomnia and nothing has worked, your doctor may prescribe sleep aids. In a recent study at the Henry Ford Health Sciences Center in Detroit, 20% of those surveyed reported taking medication, mostly over-the-counter varieties, to improve sleep.

    But before considering sleep aids, see your physician. Your doctor should determine your diagnosis, medical condition, age, and your use of alcohol or drugs before prescribing medication to help you sleep. Prescription sleep medications are available in shorter- and longer-acting forms. The shorter-acting drugs promote better-quality sleep but may wear off quickly. The longer-acting drugs maintain sleep throughout the night but may make you feel tired the next day. Most prescription sleep aids are called benzodiazepines. When taken in high doses, these medications may increase the risk of rebound insomnia, which occurs when you stop taking the drug. This will cause your insomnia to return worse than before. The best way to discontinue prescription sleep aids is to work with your physician on gradually tapering the dose.

    A new prescription medication used to treat insomnia called zaleplon (brand name Sonata) helps improve sleep without causing drowsiness, memory loss, difficulty concentrating, or lack of motor skills the next day. Zaleplon is a nonbenzodiazepine that is eliminated from the body quickly and therefore has very few next-day side effects.
- Avoid taking prescription sleep aids if you drink alcohol or if you have to operate machinery shortly after awakening, since they may cause daytime sleepiness, thereby increasing your risk for an accident. You should avoid such medications if you have sleep apnea, since the drugs can further impair your breathing.
- If depression is the cause of your insomnia, your doctor may prescribe an antidepressant medication. If anxiety is keeping you

awake, you may need to take an antianxiety drug. You will need to work closely with your doctor, since some antidepressants (especially tricyclic antidepressants) lead to insomnia or may exacerbate restless legs syndrome and period limb movement disorder.

- Over-the-counter sleep aids containing allergy medications can help make you drowsy. While these medications may be less effective and undergo less rigorous testing than prescription drugs, they have been found to be safe when used according to their directions. Avoid nonprescription sleep aids if you have respiratory problems—such as chronic bronchitis—glaucoma, or are pregnant or nursing.

- Try natural sleep remedies. Some natural remedies for insomnia include kava-kava, valerian, and melatonin. All of these have sedating effects. Five-hydroxytryptophan (5-HTP), the precursor to serotonin, is also used to promote a restful sleep. I frequently recommend 1–3 mg of melatonin or 25–50 mg of 5-HTP to my patients as an initial supplement to other sleep hygiene practices outlined above. But more is not always better, so dosage must be strictly adhered to. Care must also be taken to avoid any interactions with other natural or prescription products you may be using. Purchase natural supplements produced only by manufacturers you are familiar with. This is important because, as I mentioned in chapter 5, nutritional supplements are not held to the same rigorous standards as FDA-approved medications. There is no governing body making sure that the product meets acceptable standards for ingredients, strength, and purity. Seek the advice of a health care provider or refer to the resource section of this book to help you find reputable sources of natural health care products.

Epilogue

In 1983 *Time* magazine devoted an entire issue to "Stress—The Epidemic of the 80s." Twenty years later that epidemic has grown. Stress affects us at an even greater rate, with more pronounced effects.

I know of no greater common denominator to our ill health than the body's attempt to respond to chronic levels of excessive stress. As I've shown you in this book, virtually every major disease—cardiovascular disease, diabetes, arthritis, obesity, even cancer—has been linked to stress through mainstream medical research.

Having successfully helped hundreds of patients over the past several years, it is apparent to me that women need The Stress Cure more than ever. As the world situation becomes more complicated and more challenging—compounding the everyday stressors that burden our thoughts and push our physical stamina to the limits—we must develop ways of confronting these ever-increasing levels of stress. To understand the biology behind the behavior is not only of paramount importance to daily functioning, it is essential to a long life of health and happiness.

The Stress Cure offers great hope, both for those who are suffering in silence and for those who can clearly articulate their feelings of being overwhelmed.

I recommend that you share The Stress Cure with your health care provider. In the appendix section of this book, I've provided a letter that explains the basics of DHEA and stress reduction. You can use it to start a conversation with your medical provider that will lead to better treatment of your own condition. You may also discover that your health care professional is as stressed as you are. In that case, you may be able to follow the recommendations together and share the healing results.

The Stress Cure can help you and others in ways that have so far been overlooked by the medical profession. Use The Stress Cure to maximize your health and well-being and to live life to the fullest.

I wish you a successful journey.

Appendixes

Resources

An Informational Letter for Your Health Care Provider

Dear Doctor:

As you know, stress is a common denominator and causal agent in many of the medical conditions that affect our patients.

Your patient has just read my book *The Stress Cure* (HarperCollins Publishers). The book explains the adrenal response to the chronic and sustained levels of stress to which our patients are being exposed at epidemic levels. It reveals the basic biochemistry of the cascade of events that occur as the adrenal glands pump out cortisol to fight our internal "war of living." Sustained cortisol levels and the resultant decreased levels of estrogen, progesterone, testosterone, and dehydroepiandrosterone (DHEA) are associated with chronic stress. DHEA, a hormone derivative of cholesterol, lies at a fork in the road after cholesterol is converted to pergnenolone. The body has the choice to covert pregnenolone into cortisol—to fight the fires of daily living—or to DHEA, which it ultimately converts to testosterone and estrogens.

What I have found in my practice, which is clinically consistent with hundreds of documented research findings relating to DHEA, is that DHEA is not just a stepping-stone prohormone but also has inherent biological activity. I have found it to be a core "coping hormone," increasing our ability to cope with the daily stresses and frustrations that are cast upon us.

DHEA suffers from having been a fad hormone in the '90s. Many were taking this natural supplement without regard to proper dosages and without much knowledge of the biology of DHEA. Many health clubs used it as a way to increase testosterone and ultimately muscle. This has clouded the accurate portrayal of DHEA and left many physicians and health care providers disinclined to recommend DHEA supplementation.

I have asked your patient to share this letter with you because he or she has most likely been suffering from a constellation of stress-related symptoms. These symptoms cross over many diagnostic areas but have a common source of instigation: stress. Having documented DHEA-S and related hormone levels on over 2,000 patients in my clinic, I can tell you that there is a clear association with stress and inadequate DHEA levels. Low to nonexistent levels of DHEA cause a biologically driven behavior change. Depression, anxiety, and feelings of being constantly overwhelmed and unable to cope are symptoms of subnormal and inadequate levels of DHEA. PMS, premenopausal, perimenopausal, and menopausal symptoms are closely related to low levels of DHEA. Low libido and an inadequate sexual response can be traced to low testosterone, resulting from inadequate precursor—again DHEA.

This letter is not meant to educate you in full about the physiology and benefits of DHEA. Rather, it is a personal request from your patient and myself that you take the time to be open to learning about DHEA and to review the published literature with a medically critical eye. Be skeptical; I was initially. But give this science the professional respect that you would any other treatment or medical discovery. The bibliography and reference sections of *The Stress Cure* cite books and articles from respected physicians and medical institutions regarding the latest research pertaining to DHEA and its active metabolites.

I cannot impress on you enough what a pleasure it has been to offer a natural treatment approach that has been consistently effective and reproducible in a majority of patients.

Thank you for taking the time to review this letter. I wish you good health in this era of high stress.

Vern S. Cherewatnenko, M.D., M.Ed.

Where to Buy DHEA Supplements

At the time that I am writing this book, the following supplements are available. Before you buy, here are some points to consider:

- I recommend DHEA products that do not contain calcium carbonate as an additive. Numerous patients taking that form of the supplement report that it has not worked to their satisfaction.
- Some of the products listed are available only through licensed health care practitioners.
- You should take only DHEA that is at least 98% pure, indicating that it is of a professional or pharmaceutical grade.
- Supplements containing the raw ingredients for DHEA, *Dioscorea* yam, *cannot* be metabolized by the body to DHEA.
- Prices can vary widely among the various manufacturers.
- Consider both the milligrams per tablet and the capsules or tablets per bottle when comparing value.
- Lastly, be aware that there are some products that contain DHEA mixed with other supplements. For example, I formulated StressFree™ as a product containing DHEA along with tyrosine (to aid in increasing production of norepinephrine and dopamine for increased energy) and Saint-John's-wort (to help increase serotonin levels that moderate depression and anxiety).

The products that I have personally selected to offer in our clinic and via mail order or the Internet are listed first. The products that are available in various chain stores are listed next. There are also abundant sources of DHEA on the Internet.

When it comes to purchasing DHEA, my best recommendation is Buyer beware. DHEA products are not all created equal, and it is best to purchase them from a reputable source.

DHEA products available from Health*Max*, Incorporated:
   (I would like you to know that Health*Max*, Incorporated is my clinic and medical wellness company and I have a financial interest in the ownership of Health-*Max*, Incorporated.)

Health*Max*, Incorporated
   Valley Medical Dental Center—Suite 314
   Renton, Washington 98055
   206-362-1111
   www.healthmax.net

Products are listed in the following order:
Product Name
Manufacturer
Ingredients
Amount per bottle
Cost (at time of writing)

DHEA 25 mg
PhysioLogics
DHEA 25 mg
90 capsules per bottle
$13.00

DHEA 25 mg Sublingual Tablets
Douglas Laboratories
DHEA 25 mg
120 tablets per bottle
$15.00

DHEA 5 mg Sublingual Tablets
Douglas Laboratories
DHEA 5 mg
100 tablets per bottle
$9.00

DHEA 50 mg Capsules
AMNI
DHEA 50 mg
100 capsules per bottle
$15.00

DHEA Plus
Health*Max* via Douglas Laboratories
DHEA 25 mg and pregnenolone 25 mg
100 capsules per bottle
$15.00

7-keto DHEA
PhysioLogics
7-keto DHEA 25 mg (does not metabolize into sex hormones)
90 softgels per bottle
$25.00

StressFree™
HealthMax via Douglas Laboratories
DHEA 10 mg, L-tyrosine 50 mg, standardized Saint-John's-wort 30 mg,
vitamin B_{12} 30 mcg, Vitamin B_5 pantothenic acid 11.1 mg,
zinc citrate 10 mg, and standardized Korean ginseng 50 mg
90 capsules per bottle
$12.00

BioSom Liposomal DHEA Spray
Metagenics Incorporated
DHEA 5 mg per spray, stevia leaf extract 7 mg, and grapefruit seed
extract 330 mcg
85 sprays per bottle
$15.00

DHEA Liposomal Spray
Bio-Genesis Nutriceuticals, Inc.
DHEA 1.87 mg per spray
79 sprays per bottle
$15.00

5-HTP Complex
PhysioLogics
5-HTP from Griffonia extract 50 mg, valerian root 50 mg, niacin 5 mg,
vitamin B_6 5 mg, and magnesium 25 mg
120 capsules
$30.00

DHEA products available from other sources in the community:

The list below should not be interpreted as a recommendation of these products.
The following products are a sampling of DHEA resources available in stores
or via the Internet. Many of these companies are found in local communities.
Other stores may also carry DHEA-related products. Exercise caution when you
buy; make sure you obtain only high-quality products from reputable sources, or
consult a natural-oriented health care provider for advice in purchasing any
health related supplement.

WalMart

DHEA 50 mg
Amerifit Nutrition
DHEA 50 mg and vitamin C 15 mg
50 tablets per bottle
$8.84

DHEA 25 mg
Natrol
DHEA 25 mg and calcium carbonate 52 mg
180 tablets per bottle
$8.94

GNC—General Nutrition Centers

DHEA 25 Timed Release
GNC
DHEA 25 mg and dicalcium phosphate
90 tablets per bottle
$21.99

Albertsons Grocery Store

DHEA 25 mg
Nature's Valley
DHEA 25 mg
60 tablets per bottle
$5.99

DHEA 25 mg
Schiff
DHEA 25 mg, calcium carbonate 137 mg, and trans-ferric acid 1 mg
60 tablets per bottle
$5.99

Safeway Grocery Store

DHEA 25 mg
Safeway
DHEA 25 mg
60 tablets per bottle
$8.99

Seattle Super Supplements

DHEA—5 mg
Enzymatic Therapy
DHEA 5 mg
60 capsules per bottle
$4.68

DHEA—25 mg sublingual
Optimal Nutrients
DHEA 25 mg pharmaceutical grade
90 tablets per bottle
$11.21

DHEA—50 mg
Metabolic Response Modifiers
DHEA 50 mg micronized
90 vegetarian capsules per bottle
$15.99

DHEA Rejuvaplex
Anabol Naturals
DHEA 50 mg, L-glutamine 350 mg and vitamin B_{12} 50 mcg
30 capsules per bottle
$12.79

DHEA Complex
Biochem
DHEA 25 mg, blue cohosh extract 100 mg, chaste tree extract 500 mg,
vitamin B_6 10 mg, and vitamin E 25 IU
60 capsules per bottle
$11.21

7-keto DHEA
Kaizen
7-keto DHEA 50 mg
30 capsules per bottle
$15.96

DHEA Plus Body Cream
Life-Flo
DHEA 15 mg per pump, aloe vera, vitamin E, and MSM
2 oz (57 g)
$13.59

Vitamin Shoppe Online (www.vitaminshoppe.com)

DHEA Lipoceutical Spray
Nature's Plus
DHEA 12.5 mg per spray, vitamin E, and NADH complex
80 sprays per bottle
$14.44

DHEA Fuel
Twinlab
DHEA 25 mg
60 capsules per bottle
$9.71

DHEA 50 mg
Vitamin Shoppe
DHEA 50 mg
300 capsules per bottle
$35.97

DHEA 25 mg
Nature's Plus
DHEA 25 mg and bioperine 5 mg
60 capsules per bottle
$12.20

DHEA with Mexiyam
Solaray
DHEA 5 mg, Mexican yam 100 mg, Siberian ginseng 100 mg, and
bovine adrenal gland concentrate 100 mg
60 capsules per bottle
$6.79

Dr. Vern's Library: Recommended Reading

Alternative Medicine/Natural Medicine

Balch, James, and Phyllis Balch. *Prescription for Nutritional Healing*, 3rd ed. Garden City Park, NY: Avery Penguin Putnam, 2000.

Cooper, Kenneth. *Controlling Cholesterol the Natural Way*. New York: Bantam Books, 1999.

Crook, William G. *The Yeast Connection*, 3rd ed. Jackson, TN: Professional Books, 1989.

Goldberg, Burton. *Alternative Medicine, The Definitive Guide*, 2nd ed. Berkeley: Celestial Arts, 2002.

Goldman, Robert, et al. *Brain Fitness*. New York: Doubleday, 1999.

Janiger, Oscar. *A Different Kind of Healing*. New York: Putnam, 1993.

Kamen, Betty. *The Chromium Connection*. Novato, CA: Nutrition Encounter, 1994.

Kelly, Robert. *The American Academy of Family Physicians Family Health & Medical Guide*. Dallas: Word Publishing, 1996.

Klatz, Ronald, and Robert Goldman. *Stopping the Clock*. New York: Bantam Books, 1996.

Marti, James. *The Alternative Health and Medicine Encyclopedia*. Detroit: Visible Ink Press, 1995.

Murray, Michael. *The Pill Book Guide to Natural Medicines*. New York: Bantam Books, 2002.

Murray, Michael, and Joseph E. Pizzorno. *Encyclopedia of Natural Medicine*. Rocklin, CA: Prima Publishing, 1998.

Phalen, Kathleen F. *Integrative Medicine*. Boston: Journey Editions, 1998.

Ronzio, Robert A. *The Encyclopedia of Nutrition & Good Health*. New York: Facts on File, 1997.

Shealy, C. Norman. *The Complete Family Guide to Alternative Medicine*. Rockport, MA: Element Books, 1996.

Silverman, Harold M., et al. *The Vitamin Book*. New York: Bantam Books, 1999.

Time-Life Books. *The Medical Advisor: The Complete Guide to Alternative & Conventional Treatments*. Alexandria, VA: Time-Life, 1996.

Willard, Terry. *Herbs, Their Clinical Uses*. Calgary Wild Rose College of Natural Healing, 1998.

———. *Textbook of Advanced Herbology*. Calgary: Wild Rose College of Natural Healing, 1992.

DHEA

Callahan, Maureen. *DHEA: The Miracle Hormone*. New York: NAL, 1997.

Cherniske, Stephen A. *The DHEA Breakthrough*. New York: Ballantine, 1998.

Greenberg, Beverly. *The DHEA Discovery: Wonder Hormone of the 90's*. Los Angeles: Majesty Press, 1997.

Ley, Beth, and Richard Ash. *DHEA: Unlocking the Secrets to the Fountain of Youth*. Aliso Viejo, CA: BL Publications, 1997.

Pascal, Alana. *DHEA . . . The Fountain of Youth Discovered?* Malibu: Van der Kar Press, 1996.

Regelson, William. *The Superhormone Promise*. New York: Simon Schuster, 1996.

Schwartz, A. G., D. K. Fairman, and L. L. Pashko. 1990. The biological significance of dehydroepiandrosterone. In *The Biologic Role of Dehydroepiandrosterone (DHEA)*, ed. Mohammed Kalimi and William Regelson, New York: Walter de Gruyter.

Shealy, C. Norman. *DHEA: The Youth and Health Hormone*. New York: McGraw-Hill. 1996.

Walji, Hasnain. *DHEA: The Ultimate Rejuvenating Hormone*. Prescott, AZ: Hohm Press, 1996.

Diabetes/Obesity

Alterman, Seymour. *How to Control Diabetes*. New York: Ballantine, 1997.

Brand-Miller, Jennie, et al. *The New Glucose Revolution*. New York: Marlowe & Company, 2003.

Cherewatenko, Vern S., and Paul Perry. *The Diabetes Cure*. New York: Harper-Collins, 1999.

Rivas, Paul, and Richard B. Rothman. *Turn Off the Hunger Switch*. Paramus, NJ: Prentice Hall, 2002.

Ross, Julia. *The Diet Cure*. New York: Viking Penguin, 1999.

Sothern, Melinda, et. al. *Trim Kids*. New York: HarperCollins, 2001.

Whitaker, Julian M. *Reversing Diabetes*. New York: Warner Books, 1987.

Wurtman, Judith J., and Susan Suffes. *The Serotonin Solution*. New York: Fawcett Columbine, 1996.

Food Allergy/Toxicity

Braly, James. *Dangerous Grains*. New York: Putnam, 2002.

———. *Dr. Braly's Food Allergy and Nutrition Revolution*. New York: McGraw-Hill, 1992.

———. *Food Allergy Relief*. New York: McGraw-Hill, 2000.

Lyman, Howard, and Glen Merzer. *The Mad Cowboy: Plain Truth from the Cattle Rancher Who Won't Eat Meat*. New York: Simon & Schuster, 1998.

Schlosser, Eric. *Fast Food Nation*. New York: HarperCollins, 2002.

Zavik, Jeffrey. *Toxic Food Syndrome*. Fort Lauderdale: Fun Publishing, 2002.

Functional Medicine

Bland, Jeffrey S. *The 20-Day Rejuvenation Diet Program*. New York: McGraw-Hill, 1999.

Bland, Jeffrey S., and Sarah H. Benum. *Genetic Nutritioneering*. New York: McGraw-Hill, 1999.

Bland, Jeffrey S., et al. *Clinical Nutrition: A Functional Approach*. Gig Harbor, WA: Institute of Functional Medicine, 1999.

Galland, Leo. *The Four Pillars of Healing*. New York: Random House, 1997.

———. *Power Healing*. New York: Random House, 1997.

Great Smokies Diagnostic Laboratory. *Functional Assessment Resource Manual*. Asheville: Great Smokies Diagnostic Laboratory, 2000.

McCully, Kilmer S. *The Homocysteine Revolution*. New York: McGraw-Hill, 1999.

Packer, Lester. *The Antioxidant Miracle*. New York: John Wiley & Sons, 1999.

Quillin, Patrick. *Immunopower*. Tulsa: Nutrition Times Press, 1999.

Williams, Roger J. *Biochemical Individuality*. New York: McGraw-Hill, 1998.

General Medicine

Daniels, Rick. *Delmar's Manual of Laboratory and Diagnostic Tests*. Clifton Park, NY: Delmar, 2003.

Despopoulos, Agamemnon, and S. Silbernagl. Joy Wieser (translator). *Color Atlas of Physiology*. New York: Georg Thieme Verlag Stuggart, 1991.

Fauci, Anthony S., et al. *Harrison's Principles of Internal Medicine*. New York: McGraw-Hill, 1998.

Lehninger, Albert L. *Biochemistry*, 2nd ed. New York: Worth Publishers, 1979.

Ridley, Matt. *Genome: The Autobiography of a Species in 23 Chapters*. New York: HarperCollins, 1999.

Sapolsky, Robert M. *A Primate's Memoir*. New York: Simon & Schuster, Touchstone, 2001.

Stryer, Lubert. *Biochemistry*, 5th ed. San Francisco: W. H. Freeman, 2002.

Walsh, Paul. *2003 Physicians Desk Reference*. Montvale: Thompson PDR, 2003.

Psychology/Neurotransmitters

Cooper, Jack R., et al. *The Biochemical Basis of Neuropharmacology*. New York: Oxford University Press, 1978.

Goleman, Daniel. *Emotional Intelligence*. New York: Bantam Books, 1995.

Grabhorn, Lynn. *Excuse Me, Your Life Is Waiting*. Charlottesville, VA: Hampton Roads Publishing Company, 2000.

Harley, Willard F., Jr. *His Needs, Her Needs*. Grand Rapids: Fleming H. Revell, 2001.

Hay, Louise L. *You Can Heal Your Life*. Carlsbad, CA: Hay House, 1987.

Jantz, Gregory. *Becoming Strong Again*. Grand Rapids: Fleming H. Revell, 1998.

———. *Hope, Help and Healing for Eating Disorders*. New York: Waterbrook Press, 1995.

Keirsey, David West. *Please Understand Me II*. Del Mar, CA: Prometheus Nemesis, 1998.

Lazarus, Pat. *Healing the Mind the Natural Way*. New York: Putnam, 1995.

Murray, Michael. *5 HTP*. New York. Bantam Books, 1998.

Null, Gary. *The Food-Mood-Body Connection*. New York: Seven Stories Press, 2000.

Ornish, Dean. *Love and Survival: The Scientific Basis for the Healing Power of Intimacy*. New York: HarperCollins, 1998.

Pert, Candace B. *Molecules of Emotion*. New York: Simon & Schuster, Touchstone, 1999.

Ruden, Ronald A. *The Craving Brain*. New York: HarperCollins, 1997.

Sahelian, Ray. *5-HTP: Nature's Serotonin Solution*. Garden City Park, NY: Avery Books, 1998.

Stahl, Stephen M. *Essential Psychopharmacology*. New York: Cambridge University Press, 1996.

Vayda, William. *Mood Foods: The Psycho-Nutrition Guide*. Berkeley: Ulysses Press 1995.

Wurtman, Judith J., and Susan Suffes. *The Serotonin Solution*. New York: Fawcett Columbine, 1996.

Stress

Anderson, Robert. *Stress Power!* New York: Plenum Publishing, 1978.

Benson, Herbert. *The Relaxation Response*. New York: Avon Books, 1975.

Bloomfield, Harold. *Healing Anxiety Naturally*. New York: HarperCollins, 1998.

Crawford, Bill. *All Stressed Up and Nowhere to Go!* Humanics Pub Group, 2001.

Hanley, Jesse Lynn. *Tired of Being Tired*. New York: Putnam, 2001.

Ornish, Dean. *Stress, Diet, & Your Heart*. New York: Signet Books, 1982.

Pert, Candace B. *Molecules of Emotion*. New York: Simon & Schuster, Touchstone, 1999.

Powell, Trevor J. *Stress Free Living*. New York: DK Publishing, 2000.

Sapolsky, Robert M. *Why Zebras Don't Get Ulcers*. New York: W. H. Freeman, 1998.

Sauvage, Lester R. *The Open Heart: Stories of Hope, Healing, and Happiness*. Deerfield Beach: Health Communications, Inc., 1996.

Selye, Hans. *Stress without Distress*. New York: Signet Books, 1975.

Selye, Hans. *The Stress of Life*. New York: McGraw-Hill, 1956.

Sheehan, David V. *The Anxiety Disease*. New York: Bantam Books, 1983.

St. James, Elaine. *Living the Simple Life*. New York: Hyperion, 1996.

———. *Simplify Your Life*. Kansas City: Andrews McMeel, 1994.

Tanner, Ogden. *Stress*. New York: Time-Life Books—Human Behavior, 1976.

Vilet, Elizabeth. *Screaming to Be Heard*. New York: M. Evans, 2001.

Witkin, Georgia. *The Female Stress Syndrome*. New York: Newmarket Press, 1991.

———. *The Female Stress Syndrome Survival Guide*. New York: Newmarket Press, 2000.

Testosterone

Hill, Aubrey. *The Testosterone Solution*. Rocklin, CA: Prima Publishing, 1997.

Rako, Susan. *The Hormone of Desire: The Truth About Testosterone, Sexuality and Menopause*. New York: Three Rivers Press, 1996.

Thyroid

Rosenthal, Sara. *The Thyroid Sourcebook*. Los Angeles: Lowell House, 1995.

Shames, Richard L., and Karilee Halo Shames. *Thyroid Power: Ten Steps to Total Health*. New York: HarperCollins, 2002.

————. *Wilson's Thyroid Syndrome*, 4th ed. Florida: WilsonsThyroidSyndrome.com, 1996.

Wilson, E. Denis. *Doctor's Manual for Wilson's Thyroid Syndrome*, 4th ed. Florida: WilsonsThyroidSyndrome.com, 2001.

Wellness Medicine

Baker, Sydney. *The Circadian Prescription*. New York: Penguin Putnam, 2000.

Blaylock, Russell L. *Excitotoxins: The Taste That Kills*. Santa Fe: Health Press, 1994.

Dean, Ward, and John Morgenthaler. *Smart Drugs and Nutrients*. Menlo Park: Health Freedom Publications, 1991.

————. *Smart Drugs II The Next Generation*. Petaluma: Smart Publications, 1993.

Diamond, Harvey. *Fit for Life II*. New York: Warner Books, 1989.

Domar, Alice D., and Henry Dreher. *Healing Mind, Healthy Woman*. New York: Henry Holt, 1996.

Lamm, Steven, and Gerald S. Couzens. *Younger at Last*. New York: Simon & Schuster, 1997.

Liebman-Smith, Joan. *In Pursuit of Pregnancy*. New York: Newmarket Press, 1987.

Lombard, Jay, and Carl Germano. *The Brain Wellness Plan*. New York: Kensington, 1997.

Ornish, Dean. *Dr. Dean Ornish's Program for Reversing Heart Disease*. New York: Ivy Books, 1996.

Pauling, Linus. *How to Live Longer and Feel Better*. New York: Avon Books, 1986.

Phillips, Bill, and Michael D'Orso. *Body for Life*. New York: HarperCollins, 1999.

Pizzorno, Joseph E. *Total Wellness: Improve Your Health by Understanding the Body's Healing Systems*. Rocklin, CA: Prima Publishing, 1996.

Pritikin, Nathan. *The Pritikin Program for Diet and Exercise*. New York: Grosset & Dunlap, 1979.

Robbins, John. *Diet for a New America*. Walpole, NH: Stillpoint Publishing, 1987.

————. *The Food Revolution*. Berkeley: Conari Press Books, 2001.

Rollnick, Stephen, Pip Mason, and Chris Butler. *Health Behavior Change, A Guide for Practitioners*. New York: Churchill Livingston, 2000.

Weil, Andrew. *Spontaneous Healing*. New York: Alfred A. Knopf, 1995.

Wright, Jonathan V., and Lane Lenard. *Maximize Your Vitality & Potency*. Petaluma: Smart Publications, 1999.

Yanker, Gary, and Kathy Burton. *Walking Medicine*. New York: McGraw-Hill, 1990.

Multimedia References

McDougall, John. *Total Health Solution for the 21st Century, Volumes 1–6.* California: Dr. John McDougall, videocassette 2001.
Robbins, John. *Diet for a New America: Your Health, Your Planet.* KCET (Los Angeles) videocassette, 1991.
Time-Life Medical. *Rx Exercise—Stress & Anxiety.* Time-Life Medical/Patient Education Media, videocassette 1996.

Web sites

These Web site references are listed in the following format:
    HOST (author of site)
    URL address
    Topic areas

Alternative Medicine HomePage
www.pitt.edu/~cbw/altm.html
Resource for finding information relating to alternative medicine

American Association of Diabetes Educators
www.diabetesnet.com/aade.html
Diabetes education and online resources

American Association of Patients and Providers (AAPP)
www.aapp.net
Promotes access to care, affordable care, patient, choice, and medical freedom

American Diabetes Association (ADA)
www.diabetes.org
General information on treatment and prevention of diabetes

American Family Physician
www.aafp.org
General information for diabetes and other health concerns

American Heart Association
www.amhrt.org
Information from the American Heart Association

American Podiatric Medical Association (APMA)
www.apma.org
Information for healthy foot care

American Psychological Association (APA)
www.apa.com
Communicates the latest in psychological research and trends

American Society of Bariatric Physicians (ASBP)
www.asbp.org
Information and referrals for physicians treating obesity and related diseases

Association of American Physicians and Surgeons (AAPS)
www.aapsonline.org
Promotes patient knowledge about health and treatment options

BetterHealth USA
www.betterhealthusa.com
Information about food allergy blood testing and food sensitivities

Centers for Disease Control and Prevention (CDC)
www.cdc.gov/diabetes
Diabetes research information translated for public education

Children with Diabetes
www.childrenwithdiabetes.com
Online service for children and families with type 1 diabetes

Consumer Information Catalog
www.gsa.gov/staff/pa/cic/food.htm
Food and nutrition information

Diabetes Natural Treatment Approaches
www.thediabetescure.com
Dr. Cherewatenko's support Web site for *The Diabetes Cure* book

Douglas Laboratories
www.douglaslabs.com
Information relating to the Douglas Laboratories Corporation

Eli Lilly
www.lilly.com/diabetes/
General diabetes information from the Lilly Patient Education Program

Female Stress by Vern Cherewatenko, M.D., M.Ed.
www.femalestress.com
Information relating to stress and biological changes in women

Financial Stress
  www.pqihealth.com
  Information relating to financial stress and its biological effects

Food Allergy Relief
  www.drbralyallergyrelief.com
  Dr. James Braly's food allergy relief Web site

Foot and Ankle Web Index
  www.footandankle.com
  General information about healthy feet and resources for foot problems

Genomics and Genetic Testing
  www.genovations.com
  Genomic testing information for patients and health care providers

Great Smokies Diagnostic Laboratories
  www.gsdl.com
  Great Smokies Diagnostic Laboratories Web site

Health*Max***, Incorporated**
  www.healthmax.net
  Gateway to health and wellness information, programs, products, and services

ImmunoLabs
  www.immunolabs.com
  Information for health care providers about food allergy testing

Institute for Functional Medicine
  www.fxmed.com
  Information regarding the Institute for Functional Medicine

Juvenile Diabetes Foundation International (JDF)
  www.jdfcure.com
  Juvenile diabetes educational information

Kids and Stress by Vern Cherewatenko, M.D., M.Ed.
  www.kidstress.com
  Information on the biological effects from stress on children

Mad Cow Disease/Toxic Foods
  www.madcowboy.com
  Information relating to mad cow disease

Male Stress by Vern Cherewatenko, M.D., M.Ed.
www.malestress.com
Information related to stress and biological changes in men

Metagenics, Inc.
www.metagenics.com
Information on functional medicine, diabetes, and anti-aging research

National Eye Institute
www.nei.nih.gov
Information about eyes

National Institute of Diabetes and Digestive and Kidney Disease (NIDDK)
www.niddk.nih.gov
General information on diabetes and digestive and kidney diseases

National Institutes of Health
www.nih.gov
Access to the NIH and all the organizations that come under it

National Network for Health
www.nnh.org
Collaborative site for health education

The New Family Doctor by Vern Cherewatenko, M.D., M.Ed.
www.thenewfamilydoctor.com
Restoring the soul of family practice

Online Health Library
www.healthfinder.gov
health information resources site

Physiologics Incorporated
www.physiologics.com
Information related to Physiologics Incorporated

Simple*Care*
www.simplecare.com
Information on low-cost, cash-based health care resources

Stress by Vern Cherewatenko, M.D., M.Ed.
www.thestresscure.com
Information relating to the biology associated with stress

U.S. National Library of Medicine
www.nlm.nih.gov
The NIH source for detailed medical information

Vegsource
   www.vegsource.org/lyman
   A source for vegetarian and vegan information

Worldguide Health and Fitness Forum
   www.worldguide.com/Fitness/hf.html
   Information on anatomy, exercise, and strength training

World Health Organization
   www.who.ch
   Information on a variety of health topics and statistics

References

Ancoli-Israel, S., et al. 1999. Characteristics of insomnia in the United States: Results of the 1991 National Sleep Foundation Survey. *Sleep* 22, suppl 2 (May 1):S347–53.

Araghiniknam, J., S. Chung, T. Nelson-White, et al. 1996. Antioxidant activity of *Dioscorea* and dehydroepiandrosterone (DHEA) in older humans. *Life Sciences* 59:147–57.

Araneo, B. 1995. Proof-of-principle studies illustrating the unique adjuvant effects of DHEA-S in the immunization of elderly humans, dehydroepiandrosterone (DHEA) and aging. Meeting of New York Academy of Sciences, June 17–19.

Arlt, W., F. Callies, J. C. van Vlijmen, et al. 1999. Dehydroepiandrosterone replacement in women with adrenal insufficiency. *New England Journal of Medicine* 341:1013–20.

Arlt, W., H. G. Justl, E. Callies, et al. 1998. Oral dehydroepiandrosterone for adrenal androgen replacement: pharmacokinetics and peripheral conversion to androgens and estrogens in healthy young females after dexamethasone suppression. *Journal of Clinical Endocrinology and Metabolism* 83:1928–34.

Astin, J. A. 1997. Stress reduction through mindfulness meditation: Effects on psychological symptomatology, sense of control, and spiritual experience. *Psychotherapy & Psychosomatics* 66(2):97–106.

Azuma, T., Y. Nagai, T. Saito, et al. 1999. The effect of dehydroepiandrosterone sulfate administration to patients with multi-infarct dementia. *Journal of the Neurological Sciences* 162:69–73.

Barrett-Connor, E., N. J. Friedlander, and K. T. Khaw. 1990. Dehydroepiandrosterone sulfate and breast cancer risk. *Cancer Research* 50:6571–4.

Barrett-Connor, E., K. T. Khaw, and S. S. Yen. 1986. A prospective study of dehydroepiandrosterone sulfate, mortality, and cardiovascular disease. *New England Journal of Medicine* 315(24):1519–24, 11.

Barrett-Connor, E., and D. Goodman-Gruen. 1995. The epidemiology of DHEA-S and cardiovascular disease. *Annals of the New York Academy of Sciences* 774:259–70.

Barrett-Connor, E., D. von Mühlen, G. A. Laughlin, and A. Kripke. 1999. Endogenous levels of dehydroepiandrosterone sulfate, but not other sex hormones, are associated with depressed mood in older women: The Rancho Bernardo Study. *Journal of the American Geriatric Society* 47:685–91.

Bates, G. W., Jr., R. S. Egerman, E. S. Umstot, J. E. Buster, and P. R. Casson. 1995. Dehydroepiandrosterone attenuates study-induced declines in insulin sensitivity in postmenopausal women. *Annals of the New York Academy of Sciences* 774:291–3.

Baulieu, E. E., G. Thomas, S. Legrain, et al. 2000. Dehydroepiandrosterone (DHEA), DHEA sulfate, and aging: Contribution of the DHEA Age Study to a sociobiomedical issue. *Proceedings of the National Academy of Sciences of the United States of America* 97:4279–84.

Beer, N. A., D. I. Jakubowicz, D. W. Matt, R. M. Beer, J. E. Nestler. 1996. Dehydroepiandrosterone reduces plasma plasminogen activator inhibitor type1 and tissue plasma activator antigen in men. *The American Journal of Medical Sciences* 311(5):205–10.

Bellido, T., R. L. Jilka, and B. F. Boyce. 1995. Regulation of interleukin-6, osteoclastogenesis, and bone mass by androgens: The role of the androgen receptor. *The Journal Clinical Investigation* 95:2886–95.

Bernstein, L., R. K. Ross, M. C. Pike, et al. 1990. Hormone levels in older women: A study of post-menopausal breast cancer patients and healthy population controls. *British Journal of Cancer* 61:298–302.

Berrino, F., P. Muti, A. Micheli, et al. 1996. Serum sex hormone levels after menopause and subsequent breast cancer. *Journal of the National Cancer Institute* 88:291–6.

Berton, E., D. Hoover, H. Fein, R. Galloway, and R. Smallridge. 1995. Adaptation to chronic stress in military trainees: Adrenal androgens, testosterone, glucocorticoids, IGF-1 and immune function, dehydroepiandrosterone (DHEA) and aging. *New York Academy of Sciences Meeting* June 17–19.

Birkenhager-Gillesse, E. G., J. Derksen, and A. M. Lagaay. 1994. Dehydroepiandrosterone sulphate (DHEAS) in the oldest old, aged 85 and over. *Annals of the New York Academy of Sciences* 719:543–52.

Blissitt, P. A. 2001. Sleep, memory, and learning. *Journal of Neuroscience Nursing* 33(4):208–15.

Bloch, M., P. J. Schmidt, M. A. Danaceau, et al. 1999. Dehydroepiandrosterone treatment of midlife dysthymia. *Biological Psychiatry* 45:1533–41.

Blumenthal, J. A., et al. 2002. Usefulness of psychosocial treatment of mental stress-induced myocardial ischemia in men. *American Journal of Cardiology* 89(2):164–8.

Bobyleva, V., M. Bellei, N. Kneer, and Lardy H. 1997. The effects of the ergosteroid 7-oxo-dehydroepiandrosterone on mitochondrial membrane potential: Possible relationship to thermogenesis. *Archive of Biochemistry and Biophysics* 341:122–8.

Bonaiuti, D. 2002. Exercise for preventing and treating osteoporosis in postmenopausal women. *Cochrane Database of Systematic Reviews* 3:CD000333.

Bowers, L. D. 1999. Oral dehydroepiandrosterone supplementation can increase the testosterone/epitestosterone ratio. *Clinical Chemistry* 45:295–6.

Bremner, J. D., et al. 1998. The effects of stress on memory and the hippocampus throughout the life cycle: Implications for childhood development and aging. *Development & Psychopathology* 10(4):871–85.

Buffington, R. D., G. Pourmotabbed and A. E. Kitabachi. 1993. Case report: Amelioration of insulin resistance in diabetes with dehydroepiandrosterone. *American Journal of Medical Science* 306:320–4.

Bulbrook, R. D., J. L. Hayward, and C. C. Spicer. 1962. Abnormal excretion of urinary steroids by women with early breast cancer. *Lancet* 2:1238–40.

———. 1971. Relation between urinary androgen and corticoid excretion and subsequent breast cancer. *Lancet* 2:395–98.

Buster, J. E., P. R. Casson, A. B. Straughn, D. Dale, E. S. Umsot, N. Chiamori, and G. E. Abraham. 1992. Postmenopausal steroid replacement with micronized dehydroepiandrosterone: Preliminary oral bioavailability and dose proportionality studies. *American Journal of Obstetrics and Gynecology* 166:1163–70.

Byrne, H. K., et al. 2001. The effects of a 20-week exercise training program on resting metabolic rate in previously sedentary, moderately obese women. *International Journal of Sport Nutrition & Exercise Metabolism* 11(1):15–31.

Casson, P. R., R. N. Anderson, and H. G. Herrod. 1993. Oral dehydroepiandrosterone in physiologic doses modulates immune function in postmenopausal women. *American Journal of Obstetrics and Gynecology* 169:1536–9.

Casson, P. R., N. Santoro, K. Elkind-Hirsch, et al. 1998. Postmenopausal dehydroepiandrosterone administration increases free insulin-like growth factor-I and decreases high-density lipoprotein: A six-month trial. *Fertility and Sterility* 70:107–10.

Castillo-Richmond, A., et al. 2000. Effects of stress reduction on carotid atherosclerosis in hypertensive African Americans. *Stroke* 31(3):568–73.

Chandra, R. K. 1997. Five-year follow-up of high-risk infants with family history of allergy who were exclusively breastfed or fed partial whey hydrolysate, soy and conventional cow's milk formulas. *Journal of Pediatric Gastroenterology and Nutrition*.

Chen, T. T., et al. 1977. Prevention of obesity in Avy/a mice by dehydroepiandrosterone. *Lipids* 12:409–13.

Cleary, M. P., and J. F. Fisk. 1986. Anti-obesity effect of two different levels of dehydroepiandrosterone in lean and obese middle-aged female Zucker rats. *International Journal of Obesity* 10(3):193–204.

Coleman, D. L., E. H. Leiter, and N. Applezweig. 1984. Therapeutic effects of dehydroepiandrosterone metabolites in diabetes mutant mice. *Endocrinology* 115:239–43.

Coleman, D. L., E. H. Leiter, and R. W. Schweizer. 1982. Therapeutic effects of dehydroepiandrosterone (DHEA) in diabetic mice. *Diabetes* 31:830–33.

Coleman, D. L., R. W. Schweizer, and E. H. Leiter. 1984. Effect of genetic background on the therapeutic effects of dehydroepiandrosterone (DHEA) in diabetes-obesity mutants and in aged normal mice. *Diabetes* 33:26–32.

Colker, C. M., G. C. Torina, M. A. Swain, and D. S. Kalman. 1999. Double-blind study evaluating the effects of exercise plus 3-acetyl-7-oxo-dehydroepiandrosterone on body composition and the endocrine system in overweight adults. *Journal of Exercise Physiology Online* 2(4): 120–127.

Coyle, E. F. Physical activity as a metabolic stressor. 2000. *American Journal of Clinical Nutrition* 72(2 suppl):512S–520S.

Danenberg, H. D., G. Alpert, S. Lustig, and D. Ben-Nathan. 1992. Dehydroepiandrosterone protects mice from endotoxin toxicity and reduces tumor necrosis factor production. *Antimicrobiol Agents and Chemotherapy* 36:2275–9.

Danenberg, H. D., A. Ben-Yehuda, Z. Kakay-Rones, and G. Friedman. 1995. Dehydroepiandrosterone (DHEA) treatment reverses the impaired immune response of old mice to influenza vaccination and protects from influenza infection. *Vaccine* 13(15):1445–8.

Davidson, M. H., C. E. Weeks, H. Lardy, et al. 1998. Safety and endocrine effects of 3-acetyl-7-oxo DHEA (7-keto DHEA). *The FASEB Journal* 12:A4429.

De Becker, P., K. De Meirleir, E. Joos, et al. 1999. Dehydroepiandorsterone (DHEA) response to i.v. ACTH in patients with chronic fatigue syndrome. *Hormone and Metabolic Research* 31:18–21.

Deckro, J. P., et al. 1993. Clinical application of the relaxation response in women's health. *AWHONNS Clinical Issues in Perinatal & Women's Health Nursing* 4(2):311–9.

Denti, L., G. Pasolini, L. Sanfelici, F. Ablondi, M. Freddi, R. Benedetti, and G. Valenti. 1997. Effects of aging on dehydroepiandrosterone sulfate in relation to fasting insulin levels and body composition assessed by bioimpedance analysis. *Metabolism* 46:826–32.

M. G. Forest. 1976. Unconjugated DHEA plasma levels in normal subjects from birth to adolescence in humans. *The Journal of Clinical Endocrinology and Metabolism* 43:982–90.

————. 1978. Pattern of plasma dehydroepiandrosterone sulfate levels in humans from birth to adulthood: Evidence for testicular production. *The Journal of Clinical Endocrinology and Metabolism* 47:572–77.

Diamond, P., L. Cusan, J. L. Gomez, A. Belanger, and F. Labrie. 1996. Metabolic effects of 12 month percutaneous dehydroepiandrosterone replacement therapy in postmenopausal women. *Journal of Endocrinology* 150:S43–S50.

Dixon, Hamilton S. 2000. Treatment of delayed food allergy based on specific immunoglobulin G RAST testing. *Otolaryngology Head and Neck Surgery* 123 (1 pt 1):48–54.

Domar, A. D., et al. 1990. The mind/body program for infertility: A new behavioral treatment approach for women with infertility. *Fertility & Sterility* 53(2):246–9.

Dorgan, J. F., C. Longcope, H. E. Stephenson, et al. 1996. Relation of prediagnostic serum estrogen and androgen levels to breast cancer risk. *Cancer Epidemiology, Biomarkers, and Prevention* 5:533–9.

Dorrian, J., et al. 2000. The ability to self-monitor performance when fatigued. *Journal of Sleep Research* 9(2):137–144.

————. et al. 2001a. Increased cerebral response during a divided attention task following sleep deprivation. *Journal of Sleep Research* 10(2):85–92.

————. 2001b. The effects of total sleep deprivation on cerebral responses to cognitive performance. *Neuropsychopharmacology* 25(5suppl):S68–73.

Dunn, P. J., C. B. Mahood, J. F. Speed, and D. R. Jury. 1984. Dehydroepiandrosterone sulphate concentrations in asthmatic patients: Pilot study. *New Zealand Medical Journal* 97:805–8.

Ebeling, P., and V. A. Koivisto. 1994. Physiological importance of dehydroepiandrosterone. *Lancet* 343:1479–81.

Epstein, L. H. 2001 Reducing sedentary behavior: Role in modifying physical activity. *Exercise & Sports Sciences Reviews* 29(3):103–8.

Fenster, Laura. 1999. Psychologic stress in the workplace and spontaneous abortion. *American Journal of Epidemiology* 149(2):127–34.

Ferrando, S. I., J. G. Rabkin, and L. Poretsky. 1999. Dehydroepiandrosterone sulfate (DHEAS) and testosterone: Relation to HIV illness stage and progression over one year. *Journal of Acquired Immune Deficiency Syndrome* 22:146–54.

Findlay, E. M., M. S. Morton and S. J. Gaskell. 1982. Identification and quantification of dehydroepiandrosterone sulfate in saliva. *Steroids* 39:63–71.

Flynn, M. A., D. Weaver-Osterholtz, K. L. Sharpe-Timms, et al. 1999. Dehydroepiandrosterone replacement in aging humans. *Journal of Clinical Endocrinology and Metabolism* 84:1527–33.

Gaby, A. R. 1996. Dehydroepiandrosterone: Biological effects and clinical significance. *Alternative Medicine Review* 1:60–9 [review].

————. 1997. Research review. *Nutritional Healing* Jun: 8.

Gannon, L. 1988. The potential role of exercise in the alleviation of menstrual disorders and menopausal symptoms: A theoretical synthesis of recent research. *Women & Health* 14(2): 105–27.

Garrett, I. R., B. F. Boyce, R. O. C. Oreffo, et al. 1990. Oxygen-derived free radicals stimulate osteoclastic bone resorption in rodent bone in vitro and in vivo. *The Journal of Clinical Investigation* 85: 632–639.

Gebre-Medhin, G., E. S. Husebye, H. Mallmin, et al. 2000. Oral dehydroepiandrosterone (DHEA) replacement therapy in women with Addison's disease. *Clinical Endocrinology (Oxf)* 52:775–80.

Glaser, J. L., J. L. Brind, J. H. Vogelman, M. J. Eisner, M. C. Dillbeck, R. K. Willace, D. Chopra and N. Orentreich. 1992. Elevated serum dehydroepiandrosterone sulfate levels in practitioners of Transcendental Meditation—TM. *Journal of Behavioral Medicine* 15(4):327–41.

Gold, P. W., et al. 2002. Organization of the stress system and its dysregulation in melancholic and atypical depression: High vs. low CRH/NE states. *Molecular Psychiatry* 7(3):254–75.

Goodale, I. L., et al. 1990. Alleviation of premenstrual syndrome symptoms with the relaxation response. *Obstetrics & Gynecology* 75(4): 649–55.

Gordon, G. B., T. L. Bush, K. J. Helzlsouer, et al. 1990. Relationship of serum levels of dehydroepiandrosterone and dehydroepiandrosterone sulfate to the risk of developing postmenopausal breast cancer. *Cancer Research* 50:3859.

Hall, G. M., L. A. Perry, and T. D. Spector. 1993. Depressed levels of dehydroepiandrosterone sulphate in postmenopausal women with rheumatoid arthritis but no relation with axial bone density. *Annals of Rheumatic Diseases* 52:211–4.

Hankinson, S. E., W. C. Willett, J. E. Manson, et al. 1998. Plasma sex steroid hormone levels and risk of breast cancer in postmenopausal women. *Journal of the National Cancer Institute* 90:1292–9.

Hartke, J. R. 1999. Preclinical development of agents for the treatment of osteoporosis. *Toxicological Pathology* 27(1):143–7.

Hautanen, A., M. Manttari, V. Manninen, et al. 1994. Adrenal androgens and testosterone as coronary risk factors in the Helsinki Heart Study. *Atherosclerosis* 105:191–200.

Healey, E. S., et al. 1981. Onset of insomnia: Role of life-stress events. *Psychosomatic Medicine* 43(5):439–51.

Healey, Bernadine. 1995. *A New Prescription for Women's Health.* New York: Viking Press.

Heikkila, R., K. Aho, M. Heliovaara, et al. 1998. Serum androgen-anabolic hormones and the risk of rheumatoid arthritis. *Annals of Rheumatic Diseases* 57:281–5.

Heinonen, P. K., T. Koivula, and P. Pystynen. 1987. Decreased serum level of dehydroepiandrosterone sulfate in postmenopausal women with ovarian cancer. *Gynecological and Obstetric Investigations* 23:271–4.

Heinz, A., H. Weingartner, D. George, et al. 1999. Severity of depression in abstinent alcoholics is associated with monoamine metabolites and dehydroepiandrosterone-sulfate concentrations. *Psychiatry Research* 89:97–106.

Helzlsouer, K. J., A. J. Alberg, G. B. Gordon, et al. 1995. Serum gonadotropins and steroid hormones and the development of ovarian cancer. *Journal of the American Medical Association* 274:1926–30.

Helzlsouer, K. J., G. B. Gordon, A. J. Alberg, et al. 1992. Relationship of prediagnostic serum levels of dehydroepiandrosterone and dehydroepiandrosterone sulfate to the risk of developing premenopausal breast cancer. *Cancer Research* 52:1–4.

Henwood, S. M., C. E. Weeks, H. Lardy. 1999. An escalating dose oral gavage study of 3beta-acetoxyandrost-5-ene-7, 17-dione (7-oxo-DHEA-acetate) in rhesus monkeys. *Biochemical and Biophysical Research Communications* 254:124–6.

Herrington, D. M. 1995. Dehydroepiandrosterone and coronary atherosclerosis. *Annals of the New York Academy of Sciences* 774:271–80.

Heuser, I., M. Deuschle, P. Luppa, et al. 1998. Increased diurnal plasma concentrations of dehydroepiandrosterone in depressed patients. *Journal of Clinical Endocrinology and Metabolism* 83:3130–3.

Hillen, T., A. Lun, F. M. Reischies, et al. 2000. DHEA-S plasma levels and incidence of Alzheimer's disease. *Biological Psychiatry* 47:161–3.

Holmes, T. H., and R. H. Rahe. 1968. The social readjustment rating scale. *Journal of Psychosomatic Research* 2:213.

Iacono, G. 1998. Persistent cow's milk protein intolerance (asthma, eczema, rhinitis) in infants: The changing faces of the same disease. *Clinical and Experimental Allergy* 28(7): 817–23.

Imadojemu, V. A., et al. 2002. Impaired vasodilators responses in obstructive sleep apnea are improved with continuous positive airway pressure therapy. *American Journal of Respiratory & Critical Care Medicine* 165(7):950–953.

Irvin, J. H., et al. 1996. The effects of relaxation response training on menopause symptoms. *Journal of Psychosomatic Obstetrics & Gynecology* 17(4):202–7.

Jesse, R. L., K. Loesser, D. M. Eich, et al. 1995. Dehydroepiandrosterone inhibits human platelet aggregation in vitro and in vivo. *Annals of the New York Academy of Sciences* 29:281–90.

Johannes, C. B., R. K. Stellato, H. A. Feldman, et al. 1999. Relation of dehydroepiandrosterone and dehydroepiandrosterone sulfate with cardiovascular disease risk factors in women: Longitudinal results from the Massachusetts Women's Health Study. *Journal of Clinical Epidemiology* 52:95–103.

Jones, J. A., A. Nguyen, M. Strab, et al. 1997. Use of DHEA in a patient with advanced prostate cancer: A case report and review. *Urology* 50:784–8.

Kalimi, M, and W. Regelson. 1990. *The Biological Role of Dehydroepiandrosterone (DHEA)* Berlin: Walter de Gruyter.

Kapur, V. K., et al. 2002. The relationship between chronically disrupted sleep and healthcare use. *Sleep* 25(3):289–296.

Khorram, O., L. Vu., and S. S. Yen. 1997. Activation of immune function by dehydroepiandrosterone (DHEA) in age-advanced men. *Journal of Gerontology* 52A(1):M1–M7.

Kiechl, S., J. Willeit, E. Bonora, et al. 2000. No association between dehydroepiandrosterone sulfate and development of atherosclerosis in a prospective population study (Bruneck Study). *Arteriosclerosis Thrombosis and Vascular Biology* 20:1094–1100.

King, A. C. 2000. Personal and environmental factors associated with physical inactivity among different racial-ethnic groups of U.S. middle-aged and older-aged women. *Health Psychology* 19(4):354–64.

Kleerekoper, M. 1998. The role of fluoride in the prevention of osteoporosis. *Endocrinology and Metabolism Clinics of North America* 27(2):441–52.

Knoferl, M. W., M. K. Angele, M. D. Diodato, M. G. Schwacha, A. Ayala, W. G. Cioffi, K. I. Bland, and I. H. Chaudry. 2002. Female sex hormones regulate macrophage function after trauma-hemorrhage and prevent increased death rate from subsequent sepsis. *Annals of Surgery* 235(1):152–61.

Kubitz, K. A., et al. 1996. The effects of acute and chronic exercise on sleep— a meta-analytic review. *Sports Medicine* 21(4):277–291.

Kümpfel, T., F. Then Bergh, E. Freiss, et al. 1999. Dehydroepiandrosterone response to the adrenocorticotropin test and the combined dexamethasone and corticotropin-releasing hormone test in patients with multiple sclerosis. *Neuroendocrinology* 70:431–8.

Kuratsune, H., K. Yamaguti, M. Sawada, et al. 1998. Dehydroepiandrosterone sulfate deficiency in chronic fatigue syndrome. *International Journal of Molecular Medicine* 1:143–6.

Labrie, F., A. Belanger, J. Simard, et al. 1995. DHEA and peripheral androgen and estrogen formation: Intracrinology. *Annals of the New York Academy of Sciences* 774:16–28.

Lahita, R. G., H. L. Bradlow, E. Ginzler, et al. 1987. Low plasma androgens in women with systemic lupus erythematosus. *Arthritis and Rheumatism* 30:241–8.

Lardy, H., S. M. Henwood, and C. E. Weeks. 1999. An acute oral gavage study of 3beta-acetoxyandrost-5-ene-7, 17-dione (7-oxo-DHEA-acetate) in rats. *Biochemical and Biophysical Research Communications* 254:120–3.

Lardy, H., N., Kneer, Y. Wei, et al. 1998. Ergosteroids. II: Biologically active metabolites and synthetic derivatives of dehydroepiandrosterone. *Steroids* 63:158–65.

Leger, D., et al. 2002. Medical and socio-professional impact of insomnia. *Sleep* 25(6):625–629.

Leproult, R., et al. 1997. Sleep loss results in an elevation of cortisol levels the next evening. *Sleep* 20(10):865–70.

Lieberman, S. 1995. An abbreviated account of some aspects of the biochemistry of DHEA. Dehydroepiandrosterone (DHEA) and Aging, Meeting of New York Academy of Sciences, June 17–19.

Loria, R. M., and D. A. Padgett. 1993. Androstenediol regulates systemic resistance against lethal infections in mice. *Annals of NY Academy of Sciences* 685:293–95.

Loria, R. M., W. Regelson, and D. A. Padgett. 1990. Immune response facilitation and resistance to virus and bacterial infections with dehydroepiandrosterone (DHEA). In *The Biologic Role of Dehydroepiandrosterone (DHEA)*, ed. Mohammed Kalimi and William Regelson, 107–130. New York: Walter de Gruyter.

Louviselli, A., P. Pisanu, E. Cossu, et al. 1994. Low levels of dehydroepiandrosterone sulfate in adult males with insulin-dependent diabetes mellitus. *Minerva Endocrinologica* 19:113–9.

Mador, J. M. 2000. Quadriceps and diaphragmatic function after exhaustive cycle exercise in the healthy elderly. *American Journal of Respiratory & Critical Care Medicine* 162(5):1760–6.

Majewska, M. D. 1995. Neuronal actions of dehydroepiandrosterone: Possible roles in brain development, aging, memory and effect. *Annals of the New York Academy of Sciences* 774:111–9.

Mandle, C. L., et al. 1996. The efficacy of relaxation response interventions with adult patients: a review of the literature. *Journal of Cardiovascular Nursing* 10(3):4–26.

Markowitz, J. S., W. H. Carson, and C. W. Jackson. 1999. Possible dihydroepiandrosterone-induced mania. *Biological Psychiatry* 45: 241–2.

Mateo, L., J. M. Nolla, M. R. Bonnin, et al. 1995. Sex hormone status and bone mineral density in men with rheumatoid arthritis. *Journal of Rheumatology* 22:1455–60.

McNeil, C. 1997. Potential drug DHEA hits snags on way to clinic. *Journal of the National Cancer Institute* 89:681–3.

Merrett, J., R. C. Peatfield, and F. Rose. 1983. Food related antibodies in headache patients. *Journal of Neurology, Neurosurgery and Psychiatry* 46(8): 738–42.

Mileva, Zh., A. Maleeva, and G. Khristov. 1990. Androstenedione, DHEA sulfate, cortisol, aldosterone and testosterone in bronchial asthma patients (in Bulgarian). *Vutreshni Bolesti* 29:84–7.

Mitchell, L. E., D. L. Sprecher, I. B. Borecki, T. Tice, P. Laskarzewski, and D. C. Rao. 1994. Evidence of an association between DHEA-S and non-fatal, premature myocardial infarction in males. *Circulation* 89:91–3.

Morales, A. J., R. H. Haubrich, J. Y. Hwang, et al. 1998. The effect of six months treatment with a 100 mg daily dose of dehydroepiandrosterone (DHEA) on circulating sex steroids, body composition and muscle strength in age-advanced men and women. *Clinical Endocrinology (Oxf)* 49:421–32.

Morales, A. I., J. J. Nolan, J. C. Nelson, and S. S. C. Yen. 1994. Effects of replacement dose of DHEA in men and women of advancing age. *The Journal of Clinical Endocrinology and Metabolism* 78:1360.

Moriyama, Y., H. Yasue, M. Yoshimura, et al. 2000. The plasma levels of dehydroepiandrosterone sulfate are decreased in patients with chronic heart failure in proportion to the severity. *The Journal of Clinical Endocrinology and Metabolism* 85:1834–40.

Mortola, J., and S. S. C. Yen. 1990. The effects of dehydroepiandrosterone on endocrine-metabolic parameters in postmenopausal women. *The Journal of Clinical Endocrinology and Metabolism* 71:695–704.

Mulder, J. W., P. H. Frissen, P. Krijnen, E. Endert, F. de Wolf, J. Goudsmit, J. G. Masterson, and J. M. Lange. 1992. Dehydroepiandrosterone as predictor for progression to AIDS in asymptomatic Human Immunodeficiency Virus infected men. *Journal of Infectious Diseases* 165(3):413–18.

Murray, T. M. 1996. Prevention and management of osteoporosis: Consensus statements from the Scientific Advisory Board of the Osteoporosis Society of Canada. *Canadian Medical Association Journal* 155(7):949–54.

Nafziger, A. N., D. M. Herrington, and T. L. Bush. 1991. Dehydroepiandrosterone and dehydroepiandrosterone sulfate: Their relation to cardiovascular disease. *Epidimiological Review* 13:267–93.

Nasman, B., T. Olsson, T. Backstrom, et al. 1991. Serum dehydroepiandrosterone sulfate in Alzheimer's disease and in multi-infarct dementia. *Biological Psychiatry* 30:684–90.

Negro-Vilar, Andres. 1993. Stress and other environmental factors affecting fertility in men and women: An overview. *Environmental Health Perspectives Supplements* #101.

Nestler, J. E., C. O. Barlasini, J. N. Clore, and W. G. Blackard. 1992. Dehydroepiandrosterone: The missing link between hyperinsulinemia and atherosclerosis? *The FASEB Journal* 6(12):3073–5.

Nestler, J. E., C. O. Barlasini, J. N. Clore, et al. 1988. Dehydroepiandrosterone reduces serum low density lipoprotein levels and body fat but does not alter insulin sensitivity in normal men. *Journal of Clinical Endocrinology and Metabolism* 66:57–61.

Netzer, N. C., et al. 2001. REM sleep and catecholamine excretion: A study in elite athletes. *European Journal of Applied Physiology & Occupational Physiology* 84(6):521–526.

Nolen-Hoeksema, Susan, Carla Grayson, and Judith Larson. 1992. Explaining the Gender Difference in Depressive Symptoms. *Journal of Personality and Social Psychology*, vol. 77, no. 5.

Nsouli, T. M. 1984 Role of food allergy in serous otitis media. *Annals of Allergy* 73(3):215–19.

Nyce, J. W., P. N. Magee, G. C. Hard, and A. G. Schwartz. 1984. Inhibition of 1, 2-dimethylhydrazine-induced colon tumorigenesis in Balb/c mice by dehydroepiandrosterone. *"Carcinogenesis* 5:57–62.

Opstad, K. 1994. Circadian rhythm of hormones is extinguished during prolonged physical stress, sleep and energy deficiency in young men. *European Journal of Endocrimology* 131(1):56–66.

Orentreich, N., J. L. Brind R. L. Rizer, and J. H. Vogelman. 1984. Age changes and sex differences in serum dehydroepiandrosterone sulfate concentrations during adulthood. *Journal of Clinical Endocrinology and Metabolism* 59:551–55.

———. 1992. Long term measurement of plasma dehydroepiandrosterone sulfate in normal men. *Journal of Clinical Endocrinology and Metabolism* 75:1002–4.

Parasrampuria, J., K. Schwartz, and R. Petesch. 1998. Quality control of dehydroepiandrosterone dietary supplement products. *Journal of the American Medical Association* 280:1565 [letter].

Pashko, L. L., and A. G. Schwartz. 1983. Effect of food restriction, dehydroepiandrosterone, or obesity on the binding of 3H-7, 12-dimethylbenz(alpha) anthracene to mouse skin DNA. *Journal of Gerontology* 38:8–12.

Pizer, Frank, and Christine O'Brien Palinski. 1980. *Coping with a Miscarriage*. New York: Dial Press.

Prestwood, K. M. 1995. Treatment of osteoporosis. *Annual Review of Medicine* 46:249–56.

Prinz, P., et al. 2001. Urinary free cortisol and sleep under baseline and stressed conditions in healthy senior women: Effects of estrogen replacement therapy. *Journal of Sleep Research* 10(1):19–26.

Rafei, A., S. Peters, N. Harris, and J. Bellani. 1989. Food allergy and food specific IgG measurement. *Annals of Allergy* 62(2):94–99.

Regelson, W. 1988. Hormone intervention: Buffer hormones or state dependency. The role of dehydroepiandrosterone (DHEA), thyroid hormone, estrogen and hypophysectomy in aging. *Annals of the New York Academy of Sciences* 521:260–273.

Regelson, W., R. Loria, and M. Kalimi. 1994. DHEA—the mother steroid. *Annals of the New York Academy of Sciences* 719:553–63.

Reich, I. L., H. Lardy, Y. Wei, et al. 1998. Ergosteroids III. Syntheses and biological activity of seco-steroids related to dehydroepiandrosterone. *Steroids* 63:542–53.

Reiter, W. J., A. Pycha, G. Schatzl, et al. 1999. Dehydroepiandrosterone in the treatment of erectile dysfunction: A prospective, double-blind randomized, placebo-controlled study. *Urology* 53:590–5.

———. 2000. Serum dehydroepiandrosterone sulfate concentrations in men with erectile dysfunction. *Urology* 55:755–8.

Reus, V. I., O. W. Wolkowitz, et al. 1993. H. Dehydroepiandrosterone (DHEA) and memory in depressed patients. *Neuropsychopharmacology* 9:66s.

Rice, T., et al. 1997. Segregation analysis of abdominal visceral fat: The Heritage Family study. *Obesity Research* 5(5):417–24.

Riggs, B. L., et al. 1996. Drug therapy for vertebral fractures in osteoporosis: Evidence that decreases in bone turnover and increases in bone mass both determine antifracture efficacy. *Bone* 18, suppl 3 (March): 197S–201S.

Robel, P., and E. E. Baulieu. 1995. Dehydroepiandrosterone (DHEA) is a neuroactive neurosteroid. *Annals of the New York Academy of Sciences* 774:82–110.

Roth, T., et al. 1999. Daytime consequences and correlates of insomnia in the United States: Results of the 1991 National Sleep Foundation survey. *Sleep* 22, suppl 2 (May 1):S354–S358.

Sahelian, R. 1997. New supplements and unknown, long-term consequences. *American Journal of Natural Medicine* 4:8 [editorial].

Sands, R., and J. Studd. 1995. Exogenous androgens in postmenopausal women. *American Journal of Medicine* 98(1A):76S–9S.

Schaefer, C., G. Friedman, B. Ettinger, et al. 1996. Dehydroepiandrosterone sulfate (DHEAS), angina, and fatal ischemic heart disease. *American Journal of Epidemiology* 143(11suppl):S69 [abstr #274].

Schenker, Joseph, Dror Meirow, and Eran Schenker. 1992. Stress and human reproduction. *European Journal of Obstetrics & Gynecology and Reproductive Biology* November: 1–8.

Schiavi, R. C., and R. T. Seagraves. 1995. The biology of sexual function. *The Psychiatric Clinics of North America* 18(1):7–23.

Schneider, L. S., M. Hinsey, and S. Lyness. 1992. Plasma dehydroepiandrosterone sulfate in Alzheimer's disease. *Biological Psychiatry* 31:205–8.

Schneider, R. H. 1998. Lower lipid peroxide levels in practitioners of the Transcendental Meditation program. *Psychosomatic Medicine* (Jan–Feb) 60(1):38–41.

Schunkert, H., H.-W., Hense, T. Andus, et al. 1999. Relation between dehydroepiandrosterone sulfate and blood pressure levels in a population-based sample. *American Journal of Hypertension* 12:1140–3.

Schwartz, A. G. 1979. Inhibition of spontaneous breast cancer formation in female C3H (Avy/a) mice by long-term treatment with dehydroepiandrosterone. *Cancer Research* 39:1129–32.

Schwartz, A. G., D. K. Fairman, and L. L. Pashko. 1990. The biological significance of dehydroepiandrosterone. In *The Biologic Role of Dehydroepiandrosterone (DHEA)*, ed. Mohammed Kalimi and William Regelson, page 5. New York: Walter de Gruyter.

Schwartz, A. G., G. C. Hard, L. Pasko, M. Abou-Gharbia, and D. Swern. 1981. Dehydroepiandrosterone: An antiobesity and anti-carcinogenic agent. *Nutrition and Cancer* 3:46–53.

Schwartz, A. G., I. Pasko, J. M. Whitcomb. 1986. Inhibition of tumor development by dehydroepiandrosterone and other related steroids. *Toxicologic Pathology* 14:357–62.

Shealy, C. N., 1978. "Total life stress and symptomatology." *Journal of Holistic Medicine* 6(2):112–129.

Shi, J. and H. Lardy. 1998. 3β-Hydroxyandrost-5-ene-7,17-dione (7-keto-DHEA) improves memory in mice. *The FASEB Journal* 12:A4427.

Smith, C. 1995. Sleep states and memory processes. *Behavioural Brain Research* 69(1–2):137–45.

Smith, C., et al. 1988. Paradoxical sleep deprivation applied two days after end of training retards learning. *Physiology & Behavior* 43(2):213–6.

———. 1996. Evidence for a paradoxical sleep windown for place learning in the Morris water maze. *Physiology & Behavior* 59(1):93–7.

———. 1997. Posttraining paradoxical sleep in rats is increased after spatial learning in the Morris water maze. *Behavioral Neurosciences* 111(6):1197–204.

Smith, C. T., et al. 1998. Brief paradoxical sleep deprivation impairs reference, but not working, memory in the radial arm maze task." *Neurobiology of Learning & Memory* 69(2):211–7.

Smith, J. C. 2002. Emotional responsiveness after low- and moderate-intensity exercise and seated rest. *Medicine & Science in Sports & Exercise* 34(7):1158–67.

Stomati, M., S. Rubino, A. Spinetti, et al. 1999. Endocrine, neuroendocrine and behavioral effects of oral dehydroepiandrosterone sulfate supplementation in postmenopausal women. *Gynecological Endocrinology* 13:15–25.

Suitters, A. I., S. Shaw, M. R. Wales, J. P. Porter, J. Leonard, R. Woodger, H. Brand, M. Bodmer, R. Foulkes. 1997. Immune enhancing effects of dehydroepiandrosterone and dehydroepiandrosterone sulfate and the role of steroid sulfatase. *Immunology* 91(2):314–21.

Sunderland, T., C. R. Merril, M. G. Harrington, et al. 1989. Reduced plasma dehydroepiandrosterone concentrations in Alzheimer's disease. *Lancet* 2:570.

Suzuki, M., A. Kanazawa, M. Hasegawa, et al. 1999. A close association between insulin resistance and dehydroepiandrosterone sulfate in subjects with essential hypertension. *Endocrinology Journal* 46:521–8.

Thomas, M., et al. 2000. Neural basis of alertness and cognitive performance impairments during sleepiness: Effects of 24 hours of sleep deprivation on waking human regional brain activity. *Journal of Sleep Research* 9(4):335–352.

Usiskin, K. S., S. Butterworth, J. N. Clore, et al. 1990. Lack of effect of dehydroepiandrosterone in obese men. *International Journal of Obesity* 14:457–63.

van Vollenhoven, R. F., E. G. Engleman, and J. L. McGuire. 1995. Dehydroepiandrosterone in systemic lupus erythematosus. *Arthritis and Rheumatism* 38:1826–31.

van Vollenhoven, R. F., L. M. Morabito, E. G. Engleman, and J. L. McGuire. 1998. Treatment of systemic lupus erythematosus with dehydroepiandrosterone: 50 patients treated up to 12 months. *Journal of Rheumatology* 25:285–9.

Vgontzas, A. N., et al. 2001. Chronic insomnia is associated with nyctohemeral activation of the hypothalamic-pituitary-adrenal axis: Clinical implications. *Journal of Clinical Endocrinology & Metabolism* 86(8):3787–94.

Vogiatzi, M. G., M. A. Boeck, E. Vlachopapadopoulou, et al. 1996. Dehydroepiandrosterone in morbidly obese adolescents: Effects on weight, body composition, lipids, and insulin resistance. *Metabolism* 45:1101–15.

Wasser, S. K., G. Sewall, and M. Soules. 1993. Psychosocial stress as a cause of infertility. *Fertility and Sterility,* vol. 59, no. 3.

Weeks, C., H. Lardy, and S. Henwood. 1998. Preclinical toxicology evaluation of 3-acetyl-7-oxo-dehydroepiandrosterone (7-keto DHEA): *The FASEB Journal* 12:A4428.

Weinstein, R. E., C. A. Lobocki, S. Gravett, et al. 1996. Decreased adrenal sex steroid in the absence of glucocorticoid suppression in postmenopausal asthmatic women. *The Journal of Allergy and Clinical Immunology* 97:1–8.

Weksler, M. E. 1996. Hormone replacement for men. *British Medical Journal* 312:859–60 [editorial].

Welle, S., R. Jozefowicz, and M. Statt. 1990. Failure of DHEA to influence energy and protein metabolism in humans. *The Journal of Clinical Endocrinology and Metabolism* 71:1259.

Williams, D. P., T. W. Boyden, R. W. Pamenter, T. G. Lohman, and S. B. Going. 1994. Relationship of body fat percentage and fat distribution with dehydroepiandrosterone sulfate in premenopausal females. *The Journal of Clinical Endocrinology and Metabolism* 77(1):80–85.

Wisniewski, T. L., C. W. Hilton, E. V. Morse, and F. Svec. 1993. The relationship of serum DHEA-S and cortisol levels to measures of immune function in human immunodeficiency virus-related illness. *The American Journal of Medical Sciences* 305(2):79–83.

Wolf, O. T., O. Neumann, D. H. Hellhammer, et al. 1997. Effects of a two-week physiological dehydroepiandrosterone substitution on cognitive performance and well-being in healthy elderly women and men. *Journal of Clinical Endocrinology and Metabolism* 82:2263–7.

Wolkowitz, O. M., V. I. Reus, and E. Robert. 1995. Antidepressant and cognition-enhancing effects of DHEA in major depression. *Anuals of the New York Academy of Sciences* 774:337–9.

———. 1997. Dehydroepiandrosterone (DHEA) treatment of depression. *Biological Psychiatry* 41:331–318.

Wolkowitz, O. M., V. I. Reus, A. Keebler, et al. 1999. Double-blind treatment of major depression with dehydroepiandrosterone. *American Journal of Psychiatry* 156:646–9.

Yanase, T., M. Fukahori, S. Taniguchi, et al. 1996. Serum dehydroepiandrosterone (DHEA) and DHEA-sulfate (DHEA-S) in Alzheimer's disease and in cerebrovascular dementia. *Endocrinology Journal* 43:119–23.

Yen, S. S., A. J. Morales, and O. Khorram. 1995. Replacement of DHEA in aging men and women. *Annal of the New York Academy of Science* 774:128–42.

Yen, T. T., J. A. Allan, D. V. Pearson, J. M. Acton, and M. M. Greenberg. 1977. Prevention of obesity in Avy/a mice by dehydroepiandrosterone. *Lipids* 12:409–13.

Young, T., et al. 2002. Epidemiology of obstructive sleep apnea—a population health perspective. *American Journal of Respiratory & Critical Care Medicine* 165(9):1217–1239.

Zeleniuch-Jacquotte, A., P. F. Bruning, J. M. Bonfrer, et al. 1997. Relation of serum levels of testosterone and dehydroepiandrosterone sulfate to risk of breast cancer in postmenopausal women. *American Journal of Epidemiology* 145:1030–8.

Zumhoff, B., J. Levin, R. S. Rosenfeld. 1981. Abnormal 24-hour mean plasma concentrations of dehydroepiandrosterone and dehydroepiandrosterone sulfate in women with primary operable breast cancer. *Cancer Research* 41:3360–3.

Index